TREATING PCOS WITH THE DASH DIET

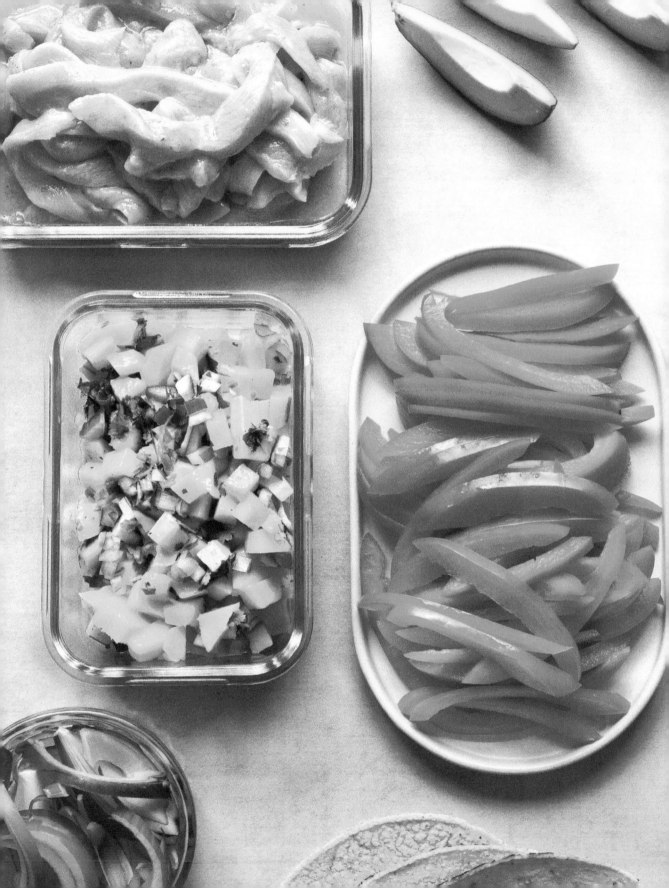

TREATING
PCOS
WITH THE DASH DIET

AMY PLANO, RD

ROCKRIDGE
PRESS

For general information on our other products and services or to obtain technical support, please contact our Customer Care Department within the United States at (866) 744-2665, or outside the United States at (510) 253-0500.

Rockridge Press publishes its books in a variety of electronic and print formats. Some content that appears in print may not be available in electronic books, and vice versa.

Interior and Cover Designer: Darren Samuel
Art Producer: Sue Smith
Editor: Marisa A. Hines
Associate Editor: Britt Bogan
Production Manager: Giraud Lorber
Production Editor: Kurt Shulenberger

Photography © Darren Muir pp. vi, 72, and Cover; © Nadine Greeff pp. ii, x, 14, 58, 60, 84, 98, 110, 122, 132, 144; © Marija Vidal, p. 30; © Jovo Jovanovic/Stocksy, p. xii; © Vera Lair/Stocksy, p. 121.

ISBN Print: 978-1-64152-717-0
eBook: 978-1-64152-718-7

This book is dedicated to all the women suffering from PCOS.

Please don't ever forget:
You are braver than you believe,
Stronger than you seem,
Smarter than you think,
And loved more than you know.

—A. A. Milne

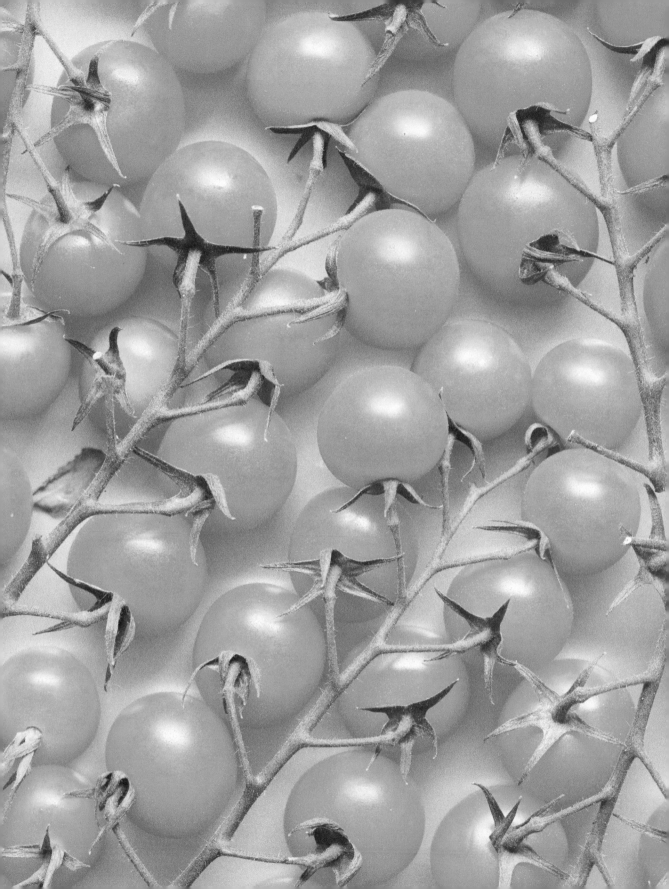

CONTENTS

INTRODUCTION

Well, hello!

I am Amy Plano, and I am a registered dietitian who specializes in the unique nutritional needs of women with polycystic ovary syndrome (PCOS). For the last 15 years I have worked closely with top specialists in women's health and reproductive medicine to learn the very best dietary and lifestyle approaches to help women with PCOS effectively manage their symptoms. Though we have much to learn about this syndrome, one undisputed fact remains clear: The driving force behind many PCOS symptoms is insulin resistance.

Although I don't suffer from PCOS, I do suffer from insulin resistance. In 2009 I began to see a significant increase in my weight. At the time, I was training for a figure competition and my diet was regimented and my workouts were diligent. Most days I was up at 4:00 a.m. to get in my training, and I was weighing, measuring, and tracking every morsel that went into my mouth.

However, despite my best efforts, I felt bloated all the time and was gaining weight, predominantly in my midsection. There are no words to describe how truly frustrated and hopeless I felt. And, to add insult to injury, I was a registered dietitian who specialized in weight loss and I could not even help myself. I felt like an absolute failure.

After trying my best to tackle this issue on my own, I decided to seek professional help. I went from doctor to doctor, only to leave having been told there was nothing wrong with me. The big problem was that, despite gaining about 30 pounds in 12 months, I was not considered overweight. So, the doctors didn't order any lab tests and chalked up my weight gain to a poor diet and not enough exercise. I am sure many of you have been in my shoes and understand just how challenging this experience can be.

But I wasn't willing to give up. I knew there had to be something else causing my weight gain. Fortunately, after much prodding from my supportive husband, we found an endocrinologist who listened to my story, took blood tests, and determined that I was, in fact, extremely insulin resistant. My insulin numbers were about four times higher than they should be for someone my size.

Fast-forward 10 years and I am happy to report my insulin levels are now under control through proper medication, diet, and exercise. However, my pre-diagnosis feelings sit heavy on my heart. There is nothing worse than believing you are doing your best but seeing no improvement in your symptoms. I have written this book for women in that situation.

Independent of medication and supplements, the dietary advice offered in this book can be helpful for any woman suffering from—or who suspects she may be suffering from—PCOS. *Treating PCOS with the DASH Diet* is aimed at women who have PCOS and who are looking for a natural, action-oriented, scientifically backed diet and lifestyle plan that can effectively decrease symptoms. This book is also written for women who have not yet been diagnosed with PCOS but who experience similar symptoms and who might be embarrassed or afraid to seek medical advice. These pages provide a clear-cut, evidence-based plan to heal your PCOS symptoms naturally.

You have heard of Dietary Approaches to Stop Hypertension (DASH), an eating program that was initially designed to lower blood pressure. DASH is more of a lifestyle than a diet. Rooted heavily in fresh fruits and vegetables, lean sources of protein, and whole grains, the diet is rich in fiber, magnesium, potassium, calcium, and antioxidants. It is low in sodium, saturated fat, cholesterol, processed foods, and sweets. All of these nutrients are critical in optimizing heart health.

Diet and lifestyle modification are, without question, the most important strategies for improving the symptoms of PCOS. The foods we eat have a direct impact on our hormones. My Modified DASH Diet for PCOS uses the DASH diet's original structure, but it controls for the overall carbohydrate content (fruits, starchy vegetables, and whole grains) with smaller serving size suggestions. Although carbohydrates are a necessary and important part of the diet, consuming too many can have a negative effect on women with PCOS. Eating whole foods that promote lower insulin levels should be the focus in a healthy diet for PCOS—and the Modified DASH Diet for PCOS has just that focus.

The Modified DASH Diet for PCOS helps control many PCOS symptoms. This eating style can help minimize insulin resistance, which can lead to major improvements in the overall health of women with PCOS or PCOS symptoms. When followed properly, the diet can promote weight loss, restore hormonal balance, and optimize insulin levels, all while decreasing a woman's risks of chronic disease.

The DASH diet has been clinically tested to decrease insulin resistance in women with PCOS. It produces measurable results not seen with other diets. Although you can't cure PCOS, you can certainly lessen its intensity to become virtually symptom free. It is my hope that you use the information in this book to improve your symptoms, prevent further medical complications, and live the very best life you possibly can. After all, girlfriend, you deserve it.

Hugs and high fives,

Amy

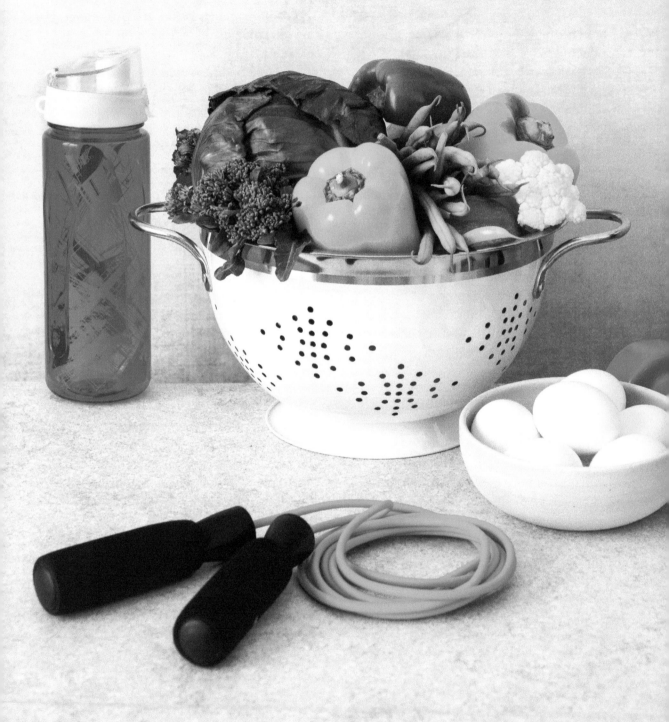

Part One

LIVING WITH PCOS

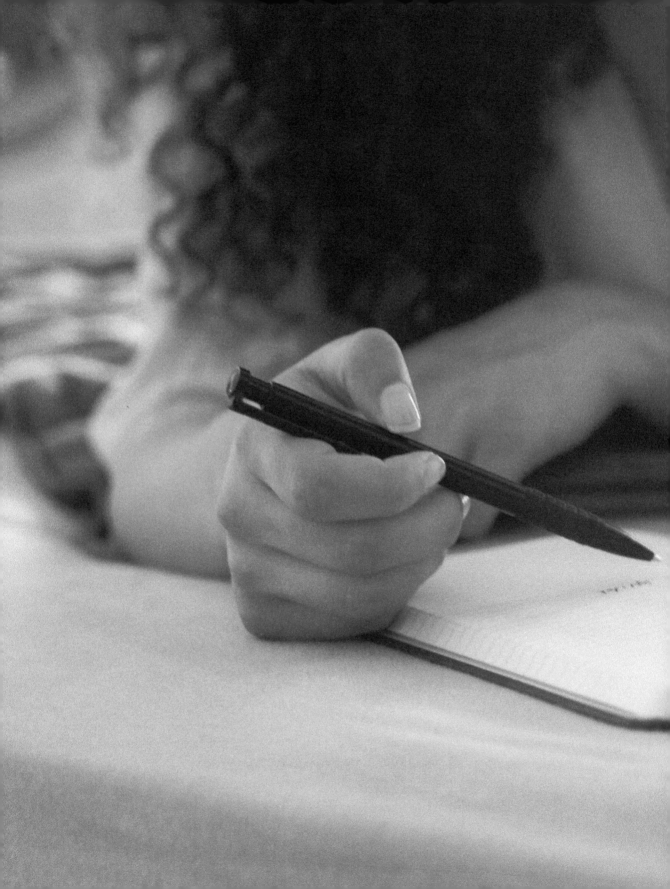

1.
UNDERSTANDING PCOS

Polycystic ovary syndrome (PCOS) is the most common hormonal disorder among reproductive-age women in the United States. PCOS can disrupt your regular periods, make becoming pregnant difficult, and it can cause unwelcome changes in your appearance. In this chapter, we explore the causes, symptoms, and inherent risks associated with PCOS. We also explore some commonly prescribed medications, methods, and supplements for alleviating PCOS symptoms.

WHAT YOU NEED TO KNOW ABOUT PCOS

There is no doubt that having PCOS can be frustrating. PCOS is a complex hormonal disorder that can be challenging to diagnose and treat. No single test can confirm whether a woman has PCOS. Instead, diagnosis is based on reported symptoms (which can vary significantly among women with the disorder), the results of blood work, and the findings from both physical and gynecological examinations. Unfortunately, many women are misdiagnosed or suffer for years without any diagnosis or proper treatment.

There is no definitive cure for PCOS. However, research supports the idea that both diet and lifestyle play important roles in controlling its symptoms. Women who change their eating patterns, exercise sensibly, and keep their stress at a manageable level have made their symptoms virtually nonexistent. The symptom management approach presented here has no unwanted side effects; you are able to get healthy *and* feel more in control of a condition that has probably been a source of great uncertainty in your life.

The first step in managing PCOS is educating yourself about the condition. The goal of this chapter is to help you confidently initiate and maintain a healthy lifestyle that decreases your symptoms and optimizes your quality of life. I am confident this information, when applied consistently, can help you take charge of your PCOS and live the life you were meant to live.

WHY DOES PCOS WREAK HAVOC ON WOMEN'S BODIES?

The symptoms of PCOS are caused by a hormonal imbalance in a woman's body. PCOS sounds like it's exclusively a disease of the ovaries, but it's not. Although this condition does indeed affect the ovaries, it's actually a full-body endocrine and metabolic disorder closely tied to insulin resistance.

Both men and women produce male hormones called androgens—just in differing amounts. Androgens play many important roles, including in hair and muscle growth, fat cell activation and storage, and libido stimulation. Blood tests show that women with PCOS secrete more male hormones (androgens) than is considered normal. This high level of androgens is commonly referred to as *hyperandrogenism.*

In women with PCOS, the majority of symptoms stem from this hyperandrogenism. High levels of androgens can:

- Cause the growth of fluid-filled ovarian cysts

- Inhibit normal metabolic patterns and promote insulin resistance

- Interfere with signals from the brain that facilitate normal ovulation

- Promote oily skin and acne

- Stimulate excessive hair growth

However, PCOS does not stop there. Women with PCOS are at increased risk of heart disease, infertility, diabetes, and obesity. They can also suffer mental turmoil brought on by the disease's symptoms. In short, PCOS can wreak havoc throughout the body.

COMMON SYMPTOMS

Truth bomb: PCOS symptoms vary among women with the condition. Some women experience only a handful of symptoms, but the majority, unfortunately, experience a heck of a lot of them in varying degrees of intensity and duration. And although these symptoms are by no means uniform, all women with PCOS experience at least some of these symptoms:

- Depression, anxiety, and sleep disturbances

- Excessive hair growth, acne on the face or torso, or both

- Intense sugar cravings

- Menstrual periods that might be absent, highly unpredictable, infrequent, or too frequent

- Oily skin

- Polycystic ovaries revealed on ultrasound

- Tendency to store excessive weight in the midsection, resulting in an apple-shaped body

- Loss or thinning of hair on the head

- Trouble becoming pregnant

- Weight issues, including weight gain or difficulty with weight loss

Because many symptoms are cosmetic, women may be less likely to report them to a health care provider. Or, they may believe the symptoms are related to a "slow metabolism" or poor family genes. As a result, many women will tolerate these symptoms for years. In fact, many women are not diagnosed with PCOS until they experience abnormal or missed periods or experience difficulty becoming pregnant.

Good news: The Modified DASH Diet for PCOS can minimize the troubling symptoms of PCOS.

Although PCOS is the most common hormonal issue for women, its precise cause is unknown. In fact, it is believed that multiple factors contribute to the development of PCOS. Research suggests that genes, in combination with certain metabolic factors, can influence a woman's chances of developing PCOS. There is a high possibility that women with PCOS inherited a predisposition for it. According to a 2007 study published in the journal *PPAR Research*, an estimated 35 percent of women with PCOS have a mother with PCOS, and an estimated 40 percent have a sister with PCOS. We have already established the strong relationship between high levels of androgens and PCOS symptoms. Therefore, any genetic defect that stimulates excessive male hormone production could be a contributing factor.

But don't run and blame your mom for everything just yet. One other critical metabolic factor that could be contributing to your PCOS is insulin resistance. We will dive deep into insulin resistance later in this chapter, but for now, just remember your PCOS is closely related to both your lifestyle and your insulin resistance.

Although you can't cure PCOS, you can lessen its intensity by managing insulin resistance. By learning how to eat better and adjust your lifestyle, you can help minimize the symptoms of PCOS and improve your fertility, reduce your risk of chronic disease, and optimize your weight.

THE CONNECTION BETWEEN INSULIN RESISTANCE AND PCOS

If you have a weight problem or can't seem to lose weight despite your best efforts, you may have insulin resistance. You are not alone. According to studies published in the journals *Human Reproduction* and *Endocrine Reviews*, insulin resistance is a key feature of both overweight and lean patients with PCOS. Therefore, to understand PCOS fully, you must develop a solid understanding of how it affects both your reproductive system and your metabolism. The hormone insulin is responsible for this connection.

HOW INSULIN CREATES PROBLEMS WITH METABOLISM

Insulin, a growth hormone, is produced by the pancreas and controls glucose (sugar) levels in the blood. Insulin's major action is to dictate how the body uses energy. Under healthy conditions, insulin levels rise briefly after eating. Insulin stimulates the liver and muscles to collect sugar from the blood and convert it to energy, causing the blood glucose level to normalize, and, in response, the insulin level as well.

FAMILY PLANNING AND FERTILITY

If you want to start a family, I have excellent news: Despite PCOS, pregnancy is possible. Making your dream come true begins with understanding how PCOS and fertility are linked.

Because a woman must ovulate to become pregnant, and ovulation is dependent on a complex balance of hormones, any disruption to that balance can hinder ovulation. Women with PCOS experience a pronounced hormonal imbalance and generally don't ovulate—which means that they cannot become pregnant.

Weight and fertility are intimately linked. Most women with PCOS are overweight. Women who don't ovulate *and* are overweight have a much lower rate of conception than women at a healthier weight. So, it is no surprise that diet and lifestyle modifications are at the forefront of fertility treatment.

Five Tips for Optimizing Fertility

1. Achieve and maintain a healthy weight.
2. Implement a natural, whole-foods approach to your diet that works to alleviate your symptoms.
3. Exercise daily.
4. Reduce stress and create a balanced life.
5. Don't lose hope—you've got this!

Many women who are trying to conceive have great success through lifestyle changes, but some need additional help. In vitro fertilization (IVF) is the most common type of reproductive technology that helps women experiencing infertility become pregnant.

IVF typically involves hormone injections to stimulate the ovaries to produce mature eggs that are then surgically retrieved. Without the help of fertility drugs, women will typically only produce one or two mature eggs each month. IVF requires lots of eggs, which then undergo fertilization in a lab, and the resulting embryos are transferred to the uterus to continue normal fetal growth. Pregnancy occurs if the embryo implants into the lining of the uterus.

Have more questions? Here are some resources and support groups that can help:

American Society for Reproductive Medicine (asrm.org): This organization is dedicated solely to reproductive medicine. Its website answers questions about infertility, IVF, and other aspects of reproductive care, diagnosis, and management.

MyPCOSteam (mypcosteam.com): This free social network for women with PCOS provides emotional support, practical advice, and personal insight on managing treatment or therapies for PCOS.

Resolve: The National Infertility Association (resolve.org): This organization offers free and low-cost programs, including referral and education programs, to help both men and women with infertility issues.

Insulin resistance occurs when the cells in your body start resisting, or ignoring, the signal that insulin is trying to send. As a result, your body becomes less sensitive to insulin and requires more of it to process blood glucose. The pancreas compensates by trying to produce more insulin. The result is a high level of circulating insulin called *hyperinsulinemia*.

Therefore, as reported in numerous studies, high insulin is not just a *symptom* of PCOS, it is also a major driver of the condition. Whereas some tissues can be resistant to the action of insulin, others, including the ovaries, remain sensitive to it. High levels of insulin can impair ovulation, causing the ovaries to overproduce androgens. These high levels of androgens are, unfortunately, responsible for the hallmark symptoms of PCOS—irregular periods, excessive hair growth, acne, and weight gain.

Women with PCOS store most of their extra weight in their midsection and often complain about their "spare tire" or "muffin top." This extra weight gain often occurs even with adequate physical activity and an appropriate caloric intake. If a woman gains weight without changing much else, excess insulin is likely the underlying reason.

More than half of women who have PCOS are overweight. Because women who are overweight are more likely to exhibit insulin resistance than those who are not overweight, elevated insulin and its resultant weight gain creates a vicious cycle. The more weight a woman gains, the more insulin is produced. The more severe the insulin resistance, the more weight she gains.

While we are discussing vicious cycles, let's also talk about the constantly fluctuating blood sugar levels that create a loop of irresistible cravings for more sugary and carbohydrate-laden food bombs. Sound familiar? It's no wonder so many women with PCOS feel hopeless, frustrated, confused, and constantly stressed.

I don't know about you, but I am so over that drama. You are not weak, powerless, or incapable of managing your PCOS symptoms. With the right lifestyle modifications, almost anyone suffering from PCOS can take control of their eating to overcome genetic influences, a faulty metabolism, and, most important, any weight issues.

Decreasing insulin levels can help alleviate many symptoms of PCOS, including hunger, cravings, and weight gain. Developing an effective strategy that lowers insulin levels and improves insulin sensitivity is the key. The Modified DASH Diet for PCOS is designed to do just that.

WHERE DOES FOOD FIT IN?

Insulin resistance makes it easy for women with PCOS to put on weight, and it makes weight loss particularly challenging. So, are there certain types of foods and nutrients that can help minimize insulin resistance, lessen PCOS symptoms, and do it all while facilitating weight loss? You bet there are! But before we dig in too deep, we need to discuss the different macronutrients supplied by the food we eat and their respective functions in the body. The three macronutrients required by the body are carbohydrates, protein, and fat. They represent energy sources and, individually, play very important roles in our bodies.

Carbohydrates

Did you know the majority of food we eat is typically made up of carbohydrates? The primary role of dietary carbohydrates is as a source of energy for the body. Carbohydrates are almost exclusively of plant origin. Milk is the only animal-derived food that contains a significant amount of carbohydrates.

There are two types of carbohydrates—simple and complex.

- Simple carbs occur naturally in foods such as milk and fruit. They are also added to processed foods, such as bakery items, frozen treats, sweet beverages, and candy, during manufacturing.

- Complex carbs are generally considered more nutrient dense as they contain fiber, vitamins, and minerals. Whole grains, legumes (beans, lentils, peas), and vegetables are all great sources of complex carbs.

In the body, simple carbohydrates break down quickly. They enter the bloodstream almost immediately, causing a rapid rise in blood sugar, which in turn triggers a rapid increase in insulin. Eating too many simple carbs can exacerbate PCOS symptoms by worsening insulin resistance and facilitating weight gain.

On the flip side, complex carbohydrates can improve insulin resistance as they slowly release glucose and allow for better insulin regulation. They also contain fiber, vitamins, minerals, and other powerhouse nutrients. Consequently, complex carbs are considered heart-healthy. Finally, thanks to their slow absorption rate, complex carbs promote an increased sense of fullness and satiety. That is why, in the Modified DASH Diet for PCOS, we place such a strong emphasis on consuming complex carbohydrates.

Protein

Protein is essential. It is required for any process in the body that involves growth or development. Your hair, skin, nails, and bones all contain protein. Your enzymes, ligaments, and hormones are all derived from sources of protein. Virtually every single cell in your body requires protein—it is *that* important! Protein mostly comes from animal foods, such as beef, poultry, pork, fish, shellfish, eggs, and dairy. Plant-based proteins include legumes, nuts, and soy.

Protein, which takes longer to digest than carbohydrates, produces a sense of satiety. Generally, protein alone doesn't require much insulin for processing because protein is not converted to glucose. As a result, protein does not raise insulin levels like carbohydrates do. We need to include protein in our meals and snacks to help stabilize blood glucose levels and to improve our overall insulin response.

Fat

You might be wondering exactly where fat fits into a healthy lifestyle for PCOS. Despite its demonization, fat is an important part of our diets. Additionally, fat supports and cushions our internal organs, helps regulate body temperature, and allows for proper absorption of several vitamins. Fat also provides the building blocks for many of our sex hormones. Fat is found in a variety of foods—from butter and oils to dairy products, meats, and processed foods.

The right types of fat, when carefully consumed, can help improve insulin levels. Like protein, dietary fat alone doesn't require insulin to be digested because it doesn't break down into glucose. An additional benefit of fat is that it helps keep us satisfied longer, thereby reducing the urge to overeat.

Despite its many awesome insulin-lowering qualities, fat cannot be eaten in any quantity you desire. In fact, diets high in certain types of fat, such as saturated fat and trans fat, can actually contribute to insulin resistance, heart disease, hypertension, and certain types of cancers.

YOU ARE IN CONTROL: THE RELATIONSHIP BETWEEN DIET AND METABOLISM

A healthy diet is the key to effectively managing PCOS. The foods we eat directly affect our hormonal systems. There is an optimal state of hormonal balance that enhances metabolism and how the body uses its fat stores. Because the underlying cause of PCOS is hormonal *imbalance*, the foods you eat can have an enormous impact on your symptoms and on the metabolic consequences of PCOS. A healthy diet, including whole foods that naturally keep insulin levels low, will be our focus here, because they are critical to controlling your metabolism and achieving long-term success.

Eating a whole foods-based diet can help stabilize blood sugar levels, minimize spikes in insulin, and balance hormone levels. A healthy diet for PCOS must:

- Be calorie appropriate to promote a decrease in body weight, as well as body fat

- Be high in fiber, vitamins, minerals, and antioxidants to decrease the risk of the chronic diseases associated with insulin resistance

- Contain a controlled amount of complex carbohydrates to regulate surges in blood glucose, minimize cravings, and lower insulin levels

- Enhance fat burning

- Have the correct balance of macronutrients to promote satiety and prevent overeating

A poor diet is not the root cause of PCOS, but it does contribute to its symptoms—and it is a factor we can control. Why wouldn't you take control of a problem when you know the outcome will be your improved health? A healthy diet should be at the top of your list of potential PCOS treatments.

COMMONLY PRESCRIBED MEDICATIONS, METHODS, AND SUPPLEMENTS

Let's look at some of the pros and cons of the most commonly prescribed solutions to treat PCOS symptoms and improve fertility.

BIRTH CONTROL

If you have PCOS, you may have been prescribed oral birth control, which can address your hormone imbalance by lowering testosterone levels. This strategy results in a more regulated menstrual cycle, which, in turn, can alleviate many of the cosmetic symptoms of PCOS, such as excessive hair growth and acne.

Birth control pills affect all women differently. It is possible you may experience mood changes, weight gain or loss, nausea, headaches, breast tenderness, and some irregular bleeding known as spotting. If your side effects are severe or don't subside within a couple of weeks, contact your health care provider, who may give you a different kind of oral contraceptive pill that may lessen your side effects.

BIOIDENTICAL HORMONE THERAPY

Bioidentical hormone therapy (BHT) has the potential to offer women with PCOS an alternative approach to balancing their hormones. Bioidentical hormones are topical treatments made from chemicals extracted from yams and soy. They are considered structurally and chemically identical to the female hormones we naturally produce in our bodies.

In women with PCOS, a lack of ovulation results in high levels of estrogen and low levels of progesterone. It is this low level of progesterone that prompts the ovaries to overproduce male hormones and that leads to irregular periods or the lack of ovulation, and, ultimately, infertility issues. BHT is applied at certain times during your cycle to help restore balance to your hormone levels.

The main concern with BHT products is their overall safety and effectiveness. They tend to be marketed as a more natural alternative to conventional hormone therapy, but no BHT products have been approved by the Food and Drug Administration. Minimal research on the use of BHT for PCOS means that the products' short- and long-term side effects are difficult to assess. In short, the potential consequences of prolonged or minimal use of BHT products are not yet fully known.

OVULATION INDUCTION

If you have PCOS, there is a good chance you don't ovulate. A method called ovulation induction, with pills or injections, may help stimulate your ovaries to increase egg production so you can become pregnant.

The first type of ovulation induction for improving fertility in women with PCOS is clomiphene, which is administered orally. The benefits of clomiphene include its low cost, ease of administration and monitoring, and remarkable success at inducing ovulation and planned pregnancies.

The side effects vary. Some women report hot flashes, mood swings, bloating, and breast tenderness as well as visual changes such as blurred vision. There is also a slightly higher risk of multiple pregnancies with clomiphene than with conventional conception.

The second type of ovulation induction is gonadotropin injections, which contain follicle-stimulating hormone alone or combined with luteinizing hormone to help produce mature eggs in the ovaries. There are two significant complications with the use of gonadotropin injections in women with PCOS. One is an increased risk of multiple births. Sometimes the drugs are almost too effective. Rather than stimulating and maturing just one egg, the ovaries respond by releasing multiple follicles (cysts containing eggs), which then creates the potential for having twins or even triplets. The second concern, though rare, is a condition called ovarian hyperstimulation syndrome (OHSS), which can occur when the ovaries become overstimulated, resulting in abdominal swelling, nausea, bloating, and, in some serious cases, chest pain and difficulty breathing. Generally, at this point, the treatment stops and other options are considered.

DIETARY SUPPLEMENTS

The use of dietary supplements to treat PCOS is an exciting and important area of study. The use of all supplements should involve a detailed assessment of your diet, and any medications and/or other supplements you may be taking. Contact your health care provider before starting any supplement use on your own.

Magnesium supplements: Studies have shown that magnesium supplementation may be beneficial for women with PCOS thanks to its ability to improve insulin resistance, blood pressure, and overall metabolic syndrome, among other things. Additionally, birth control pills can lower your magnesium levels, and supplementing with magnesium is a fairly inexpensive and natural way to address this side effect, while also improving your energy, mood, hormone balance, and bowel regularity. Keep in mind that, for some women, magnesium supplementation can cause gastrointestinal issues, such as abdominal cramping, nausea, vomiting, and diarrhea. Although rare, excessive magnesium ingestion can cause increased thirst, drowsiness, confusion, muscle weakness, respiratory depression, coma, and cardiac arrest. So, as with any supplement, speak with your health care provider first, and start with the lowest recommended amount. For magnesium, that is about 100 mg per day. The National Academy of Medicine doesn't endorse doses of more than 350 mg supplemental magnesium per day.

Myo-Inositol and D-Chiro-Inositol: Inositol naturally occurs in foods such as fruits, beans, grains, and nuts. Your body can also produce inositol from carbohydrates you eat. However, research published in the *International Journal of Endocrinology* suggests additional inositol in the form of supplements may have numerous health benefits for women with PCOS. Taking one or both of two particular forms—myo-inositol and D-chiro-inositol—can have a number of positive effects, including lowering testosterone levels, decreasing blood pressure, and improving ovarian function in overweight or obese women with PCOS. Inositol supplements appear to be well tolerated by most women, but mild side effects have been reported, including nausea, gas, difficulty sleeping, headache, dizziness, and tiredness. Whereas studies have revealed many important and useful properties of myo-inositol or D-chiro-inositol, more long-term studies are needed to determine their recommended dosages, safety, and overall effectiveness. Nevertheless, the little evidence that's currently available on inositol supplementation looks promising for women with PCOS.

THE CONTROVERSY OF BIRTH CONTROL PILLS

Birth control pills for women with PCOS is a hot topic. Although birth control pills are considered a primary treatment, along with diet and lifestyle modification, for the symptoms of PCOS, many symptomatic women are just saying "no." Let's examine the reasons many women with PCOS seek alternate options:

Unwanted side effects: The side effects may include bloating, decreased libido, weight gain, mood swings, depression, anxiety, and nausea.

Masked reproductive health issues: Some women feel birth control masks symptoms, instead of treating them, by chemically altering the hormones.

Increased risk of certain diseases: Women with PCOS who are obese and/or smoke already have an increased risk of cardiovascular diseases. Adding birth control pills to the mix further increases these risks, with a particular risk of blood clots. Your cardiovascular risk should be formally assessed before you even considering taking a birth control pill.

However, there are also numerous benefits to the pill. In addition to providing effective contraception if you are sexually active, studies have found that birth control pills can also offer protection from endometrial cancer. Birth control pills can help regulate your period and decrease your levels of androgens, which can improve many of the cosmetic side effects of PCOS, such as acne and excessive hair growth.

Whether you decide to use birth control pills is a personal decision that should be carefully made with the guidance of your health care provider. PCOS treatment should be uniquely tailored to your symptoms, other health problems, and whether you want to become pregnant.

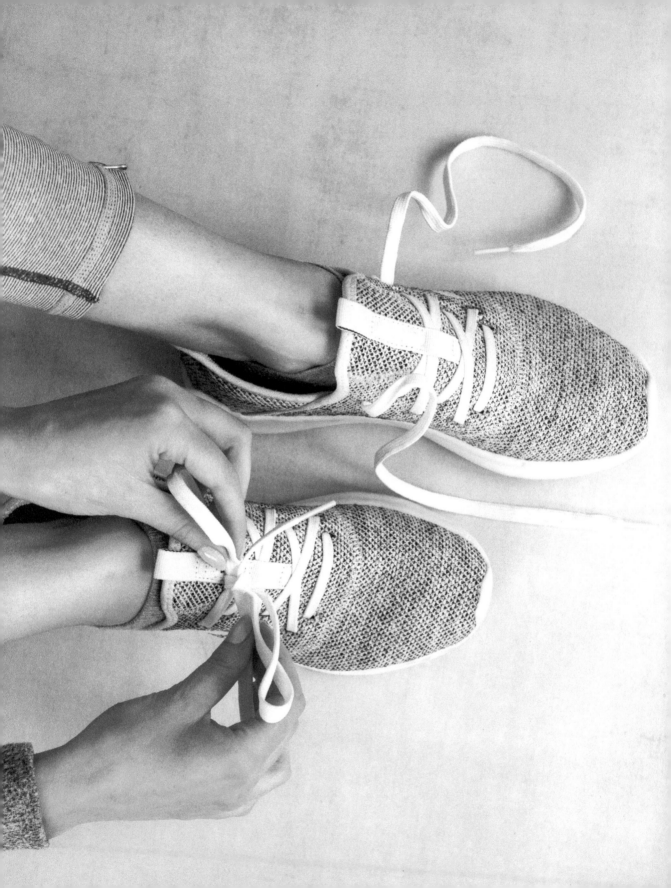

2.
THE IMPORTANCE OF A HEALTHY LIFESTYLE

Both diet and lifestyle changes are critical to managing PCOS symptoms. Getting adequate sleep and managing your stress and personal relationships are paramount when it comes to improving your overall health and well-being. Exercise not only helps you stay healthy, but also helps you feel better about that beautiful body of yours. By following a healthy diet and lifestyle you can heal the symptoms of PCOS and dramatically improve your quality of life.

SLEEP AND REST

Did you know women with PCOS are more likely to suffer from sleep disturbances than the general population? Studies support that sleep deprivation and PCOS symptoms are linked in several ways. Hormonal changes brought on by poor sleep can lead to weight gain and obesity, among other things. You certainly won't be surprised, then, that I consider sleep one of the most important pillars of PCOS symptom management.

Sleep disturbances are intimately tied to insulin resistance. It is well-documented that many women who suffer from PCOS also have insulin resistance. When you don't get enough sleep your body responds by changing the way it produces and uses insulin. As we've already learned, insulin enables the body's cells to absorb glucose from the bloodstream and use it for energy, thereby regulating blood glucose levels.

Poor-quality sleep also increases production of another hormone, cortisol. Think of cortisol as your very own alarm system. It's your body's main stress hormone. Too much cortisol makes your cells more resistant to insulin. Poor-quality sleep also prompts changes in other hormones, including your thyroid-stimulating hormone and testosterone, which means more insulin resistance and higher blood glucose levels.

Sleep also affects our appetite. When we don't get enough sleep, the hormones that regulate hunger and our feelings of fullness are affected, increasing the risk of obesity.

Although it can be difficult to get a full night's sleep, here are three awesome tips to help you get a better night's rest.

Ditch the caffeine after 2 p.m. Avoid all forms of caffeine—and sugar—well before bedtime so you are able to relax and fall asleep more easily.

Become a creature of habit. Creating good sleep patterns is important. Create a routine so your body becomes accustomed to falling asleep and waking at the same times each day.

Create an electronics-free zone in your bedroom. The blue light emitted from cell phones, tablets, and laptop screens affects our circadian rhythms. The best practice is to turn off all screen devices two hours before bedtime.

Sleep disturbances can be frustrating for everyone, but especially for women with PCOS because it contributes to the symptoms. Look for natural ways to bring on better and more regular sleep, and you'll wake knowing you're doing your best to manage your health and improve your well-being.

STRESS MANAGEMENT

You have just learned why sleep is crucial in managing PCOS. Now, you will learn how stress can affect PCOS. Though invisible, stress has a profound ability to affect both the psychological and physical aspects of women living with PCOS. Stress can affect your emotions, mood, hormones, and immune function. These factors, in turn, can affect your appetite, weight, and, ultimately, fertility.

There is no shortage of stress in our lives—from brutally long work weeks to poor sleep patterns to incessant negative feelings about our bodies and physical appearance, we are constantly bombarded from every direction. Throw in a diagnosis of PCOS, imbalanced hormones, and weight gain—despite our best efforts—and we have a recipe for a pretty stressful life.

The pituitary gland is an important player in stress response. When we are stressed, the area in the brain called the hypothalamus stimulates the pituitary gland to secrete adrenocorticotropic hormone (ACTH). In response, the adrenal glands that sit on top of the kidneys respond by producing what we refer to as "the stress hormones": cortisol, adrenaline, and noradrenaline. High circulating levels of ACTH also increase the production of androgens, which contribute to many PCOS symptoms.

When we are under stress, our bodies secrete cortisol. However, once the threat is removed, our cortisol levels should drop. Research reported in *The Journal of Clinical Endocrinology & Metabolism* showed that, regardless of weight, women with PCOS have higher levels of the stress hormone cortisol. Women with PCOS don't only secrete higher-than-normal levels of cortisol, but the hormone tends to remain elevated for a longer period. Cortisol can affect the body in many ways. High levels of cortisol can cause you to consume more calories. In other words when stress levels are high you eat more. Not only do you consume more calories when stressed, you tend to gravitate toward sweet and sugary foods.

When we experience high levels of cortisol, our body responds by releasing glucose. Unfortunately, many of us are fairly sedentary and the body doesn't need that glucose for fuel. So the body tries to get rid of the excess glucose by raising the amount of insulin it produces. However, if you have PCOS this process doesn't work like it should. Instead, the extra glucose gets stored as fat. Therefore, chronically elevated cortisol levels can result in insulin resistance or, in many cases, the worsening of insulin resistance.

High levels of cortisol can directly affect fertility by interfering with progesterone production. Cortisol and progesterone compete for the same receptor sites in the ovaries. When this tug-of-war goes on for too long, you may experience problems with your menstrual cycle and your estrogen balance, contributing to infertility issues. The imbalance of cortisol and progesterone further contributes to weight issues, skin conditions, and low energy levels, which can cause—you guessed it— more stress.

So, now that you know how stress affects your body, consider these tips for managing it:

- Maintain a healthy diet that works with your PCOS symptoms, not against them.

- Aim for at least seven to eight hours of quality sleep each night.

- Decrease your caffeine consumption.

- Surround yourself with positive, supportive people.

- Make exercise part of your daily routine.

- Set aside appropriate time each week for rest, relaxation, and/or self-care.

- Engage in consistent enjoyable stress management techniques (see next section).

STRESS MANAGEMENT TECHNIQUES

Stress management techniques, which include various forms of meditation, yoga, and Tai Chi, can play an important role for women with PCOS. Stress occurs when you feel threatened or are unable to cope with a particular situation. Yes, a little stress can actually be a good thing (Hello, motivation!), but when chronic, stress can have a huge negative effect on our health and overall well-being. According to a 2015 study by researchers at the Penn State College of Medicine, although stress management techniques can't magically make stress disappear, when practiced regularly, they can produce favorable decreases in blood pressure, blood sugar levels, and psychological distress and improve overall quality of life.

If left untreated, stressors can lead to anxiety and depression. Although meditation, yoga, and Tai Chi are all different, they all work on reducing stress in a similar way—by slowing breathing, regulating heart rate, and increasing the amount of oxygen circulating throughout your body. In addition, they center your thoughts in an effort to decrease the negative thought patterns and emotions that contribute to daily stressors. By keeping you in the present moment with your attention on current thoughts, feelings, and emotions without passing judgment, you can balance your mind and, in turn, balance your hormones.

Other stress management techniques can include:

- Keeping a positive mind-set

- Letting go of the things in life you can't control and focusing your attention on the ones you can

- Surrounding yourself with a good support system

- Eating small, frequent meals and snacks to stabilize your blood sugar and optimize your mood

- Making time in your life for the things that you enjoy, like your friends, family, hobbies, and personal interests

No matter what stress management technique you choose, engage in it regularly to experience the benefits. Choose one you think you might enjoy doing regularly and give it a go. If you find you don't love it, try another. What is most important is that you begin engaging in practices that will help manage your overall stress, and you can begin with just five minutes a day.

EXERCISING WITH PCOS

Exercise is critical to managing the symptoms of PCOS. The benefits of exercise are seemingly endless. Exercise can help:

- Manage your insulin resistance

- Enhance your mood

- Optimize your weight

- Improve sleep patterns

- Decrease your risk of chronic diseases such as diabetes, heart disease, and osteoporosis

- Help burn belly fat

Despite its numerous benefits, exercise can be difficult to incorporate into your life. In fact, if you're like some women, exercise may be one of the last things you want to do.

But what if you shifted your mind-set to see exercise as a celebration of what your body can do? Rather than forcing yourself to hit the gym in the hopes of looking thinner, what if you focused on the long-term health benefits of exercise? I know it is challenging, but try not to think of exercise as something you have to do, or should do. Instead, think of it as a way to help you feel better.

I get it. The struggle is real. Here are some tips for increasing physical activity and exercise:

Take it in stride. Starting an exercise program can be overwhelming, but it doesn't have to be. Start simple and start slow. Even small amounts of physical activity can have a big impact on your health—like a simple walk, which requires no special equipment, except maybe some sturdy shoes. Turn up the tunes, listen to a podcast, or invite a friend to join you.

Do what you enjoy. Choose fun activities you enjoy. For instance, do you like to walk around your neighborhood or hike in the woods? What about group activities, such as water aerobics or Zumba?

Schedule it. Keep your promise to yourself and schedule exercise into your weekly routine. Putting it in your calendar, like a doctor's appointment, can increase your chances of committing to your goal. You would never not show up for a doctor's appointment—not showing up for yourself is not an option either.

Get wet. Think outside the exercise box. Water workouts can be very beneficial for women with PCOS. You'll get a full-body workout that's also easy on the joints. Continuing to think outside that box, you don't always need to get *in* the water . . . try stand-up paddleboarding for a fun way to tighten, tone, and build balance awareness.

How much exercise do you need? Where is that sweet spot of consistent benefits from exercise without injuries? So glad you asked. Shoot for at least 150 minutes of moderate activity (brisk walking, heavy housecleaning) or 75 minutes of vigorous exercise (hiking, jogging, aerobic dancing) per week.

It is generally beneficial to perform a combination of both cardiovascular and strength-training exercises. However, if you are just starting out, I suggest getting in the habit of moving your body on a consistent basis. Raising your heart rate forces your body to use stored energy as fuel, which results in calorie expenditure. Research reported in the *Saudi Journal of Sports Medicine* found that cardio exercises have also been shown to lower the risk of cardiovascular disease in women with PCOS. Strength training, on the other hand, supports muscle growth, which is important in raising metabolism, improving body composition, lowering blood sugar levels, and making your body sensitive to the effects of insulin.

Some of you may be old pros when it comes to exercising, but others may not be. Guess what? That is OK. We all need to start somewhere. So, if you are new to exercise, have been sedentary for many years, have a significant amount of weight to lose, or just consider yourself out of shape, I have the perfect four-week walking program to get you started. Before beginning, though, speak with your health care provider to be cleared for exercise. If you are undergoing fertility treatments, you should also speak with your reproductive endocrinologist before starting any exercise program, as there may be times when exercise needs to be avoided during treatment.

Week One (40 Minutes): The goal for week one is to establish a habit, so consistency is important. You'll walk two days this week, 20 minutes each time, at an easy pace. If you find 20 minutes at once too challenging, break the 20 minutes into more manageable blocks of time, say two 10-minute walks or four 5-minute sessions.

Week Two (75 Minutes): You are gaining steam now. Add five minutes each day and then one more day so you are walking 25 minutes, three days this week.

Week Three (120 Minutes): You are on a roll! Add another five minutes each day, and then one more day so you are walking for 30 minutes, four days this week.

Week Four (150 Minutes): Final push. You've got this! This week keep walking for the same amount of time, but add one more day, so you are walking for 30 minutes, five days this week.

Imagine how wonderful you'll feel as you move through and hit each of these goals—and you will! Once you've completed this four-week plan, you'll be ready for a variety of different workouts to add intensity and endurance.

PERSONAL RELATIONSHIPS

Whether you are dating, in a fully committed relationship, or just hanging out with friends, PCOS can take a toll on relationships. Your hormone imbalance can make you feel not like yourself, which can leave you sad, angry, frustrated, disconnected, and lonely. Poor satisfaction with your body and low self-esteem can further complicate relationships. But there are easy actions you can take to boost your confidence and improve your emotional well-being, all while fostering the loving and rewarding relationships you deserve. Let's dive into some of the juicy details.

This whole process of dating can be strange, awkward, and downright frightening for pretty much everyone. Combine this with the cosmetic burdens of PCOS and the thought of dating can become downright unbearable. The changes to your physical appearance can lower your self-esteem, causing you to feel uncomfortable in your own body. Ready for an important truth bomb? PCOS doesn't define you. Here are three of my favorite tips for enhancing self-esteem when it comes to dating:

1. **Embrace your awesomeness.** It might sound simple, but reminding yourself of your awesome qualities is guaranteed to boost your confidence. Grab a cute journal and make a list of all your great qualities, including anything (and everything) that makes you smile about yourself. Trust me. You are going to be blown away by your awesomeness. And if you are blown away by your awesomeness, anyone you might want to date will be, too.

2. **Practice positive affirmations.** When dealing with PCOS, being told to be positive can be a little annoying. However, affirmations are an effective way to help combat your negative thoughts. These can help cultivate feelings of self-love and self-worth. Understanding your value and self-worth will inspire confidence and spark joy, growth, and authentic love, all allowing you to revel in a relationship that is kind, mutually respectful, and meaningful.

   Here are some of my favorite affirmations on relationships you can say to yourself daily: "I am happy and have everything I need," "I feel safe and comfortable in my body," and "I love and cherish who I've become."

3. **Invest in self-care.** Self-care is doing things for yourself that make you feel good. Optimal nutrition, sleep, and exercise form the foundation of self-care. All of these will help manage PCOS symptoms and can help you feel better in your own skin. No relationship is sustainable if we don't attend to our own needs first. So, give yourself the care you need and I'm certain you, and those around you, will appreciate the fantastic return on that investment.

COMMITTED RELATIONSHIPS

So, congrats! You made it past that awkward dating phase. Now let's look at some issues you may experience in a committed relationship and how they can be successfully managed.

Sharing intimacy. Opening up about your sex life to medical professionals may not only be uncomfortable, but can also place a real strain on your relationship. Being told when to have sex decreases the level of spontaneity and fun that comes with being a couple. Sex can, unfortunately, turn into a chore for those who are trying to conceive. Work with your partner to think of fun and creative ways to initiate sex. Also, make an effort to connect outside the bedroom. Finally, reassure each other that this change in your sexual relationship is only temporary.

Feeling sexy. Research reports that women with PCOS often experience a low sex drive and/or sexual dysfunction. Though doctors are unsure of the specific cause of this, they believe it is tied to the hormonal imbalances in women with PCOS. Compounding matters further, like many women with PCOS, you may feel uncomfortable during sex because of the physical and cosmetic symptoms. This discomfort can affect the ability to have an orgasm. It can also affect your overall mental well-being and attitude toward sex, which might ultimately put a strain on your relationship. But sex doesn't have to be something you avoid. It should be something you do with your partner to feel closer and more connected. Why not try engaging in activities that help you feel more comfortable and connected with yourself? Any movement-based activity, such as yoga, Pilates, or dance, can help you experience just how beautifully your body can function.

Handling the shock factor. Because so many women with irregular periods are given birth control pills at a young age, many don't actually know they have PCOS until they are in a committed relationship and trying to conceive. The pill helps decrease many of the physical symptoms of PCOS. Therefore, it is infertility that leads these women to a diagnosis of PCOS. Infertility diagnoses can leave many women feeling dejected, confused, hopeless, and riddled with guilt. Are you one of them? If so, you are not alone in your struggle. There are several medical and nonmedical interventions available to treat infertility and help you become pregnant. Deciding which option is appropriate for you will probably include a discussion with your partner and health care team. Ultimately, it is your body and you should choose what feels most comfortable.

Learning to work as a team. Many women who struggle to conceive may experience an enormous amount of guilt. They feel as if their bodies have failed them. This feeling of failure is not just from a conception perspective. Many women experience uncontrollable mood swings, depression, and anxiety—all related to their diagnosis. This behavior can easily spill out into the context of relationships. It is important to remember that talking to your partner about PCOS should be an ongoing conversation—not just something you talk about once and never discuss again. Asking for support when you need it is important and can actually strengthen your relationship. Working together regarding treatment is critical to the health of your relationship.

Understanding that maintaining a relationship can be hard. There is no doubt that you will be stronger and more emotionally healthy when you create relationships that are open, honest, and authentic. Hiding out because you're tired, moody, or embarrassed about your body only makes things worse. Understanding how PCOS affects your relationships is the first step to improving them. If you feel your relationship is suffering because of your PCOS, please consider reaching out to your doctor, a psychologist, or other licensed health care practitioner.

EATING HABITS

Food has a critical role in the PCOS saga. The food we eat has a direct effect on our hormones. Therefore, both the quality and quantity of the foods you consume can have a significant impact on your PCOS.

I would be lying to you if I told you that changing your eating patterns is easy; and the intricate involvement of both the endocrine and metabolic systems in PCOS makes changing your eating habits even more challenging. Let's examine three critical ways your eating habits can be affected by PCOS. Unsurprisingly, all three involve the hormone insulin.

Fat storage mode. As we have discussed, many women with PCOS have insulin resistance. Women with PCOS secrete too much insulin. There are two types of hormones the body produces: *anabolic* and *catabolic*. Anabolic hormones relay the message to the body to "build or store," whereas catabolic hormones tell the body to "break down" tissues and structures. Insulin is considered an anabolic hormone, as is the male hormone testosterone. In the case of PCOS, women have both. Too much insulin causes the body to store body fat and prompts weight gain—independent of one's eating habits—primarily in a woman's midsection, resembling what some women refer to as a muffin top or spare tire.

Stress mess. Both the physical and emotional aspects of PCOS can have a significant impact on your eating patterns. Excess hair growth, weight gain, menstrual irregularities, acne, and infertility are just a handful of the numerous stressors women with PCOS experience. Given the magnitude of stress women with PCOS face, it is unsurprising that there is a high prevalence of depression among these women. Though stress manifests in different ways for different people, two of the most common consequences are overeating and eating when not hungry. When people are stressed they tend to reach for foods that are comforting, like sweets and carbohydrate-dense foods. These foods only make matters worse for women with PCOS.

WHEN YOUR FRIENDS DON'T UNDERSTAND

Even though PCOS is surprisingly common, most people have never heard of it, so there is a good chance even your closest friends don't fully understand the daily difficulties you face. If your friends are not properly informed, it is easy for them to base their understanding on culturally ingrained assumptions: If you are obese, they might think you have no willpower. If you have acne, they might assume you practice poor self-care. And even if they think they have the slightest clue as to what this disorder entails, it's no surprise if they zero in on just the ovarian part. This lack of awareness is not uncommon, as the name itself doesn't even remotely explain the complex physical, energetic, and emotional aspects of PCOS.

Ultimately, when it comes to your closest friends, you are in control of what you choose to share and not share. Not everyone is ready to talk about their PCOS and all the symptoms, emotional and physical pain, and heartache that comes with it—and that is okay. However, some women report that by talking about PCOS with their friends, they experience a sense of freedom because they no longer need to hide their condition. For others, the more they talk about it the more they recognize they are not alone.

No matter what you decide, remember your friends love you for who you are, not because you have clear skin and perfect hair and are always in a good mood. They want to be friends with you because of the value you add to their life, and vice versa. Respect yourself, and trust that a true friend will be there no matter what.

Because women with PCOS suffer from insulin resistance, they don't process sugary, carbohydrate-rich foods effectively. A higher-carbohydrate meal will often cause their blood sugar to drop quickly, leaving them tired, hungry, anxious, and feeling pretty lousy overall. This blood sugar drop adds more stress and promotes a vicious cycle of what may appear to be poor eating habits, but is actually just a symptom of the disorder.

Got cravings? It has been reported that women with PCOS experience more cravings than women without PCOS. Much of this is related to the way their bodies process insulin and regulate blood sugar. Not only does insulin promote fat storage, it is also a well-known appetite stimulant. This stimulant helps explain why many women with PCOS and insulin resistance often experience intense hunger and pronounced cravings for carbohydrate-rich foods. These cravings can even occur immediately after they eat a large meal, even though they aren't really physically hungry. If not addressed, these cravings can turn into unwanted calories and weight gain.

I understand these scenarios can all be extremely frustrating—but they don't have to be. By altering your diet and lifestyle, you can control your insulin resistance and gain control of your eating habits. Let's examine the foods and eating patterns that will support your success.

WHAT HABITS TO KICK

As you are likely aware by now, lifestyle plays a significant role in PCOS. I hate to be a "Debbie Downer," but there are certain habits you need to kick. These habits are standing in the way of you feeling better and can actually be making your symptoms worse. The quicker you break up with these habits, the sooner you will be on your way to seeing positive results.

Let's start with the most obvious habits to break. Smoking and recreational drugs have no place in your journey to healing PCOS. As you've learned, PCOS increases your risk of certain diseases, among them cardiovascular issues and diabetes. Don't add fuel to the fire by continuing to make these unhealthy choices. They will not help you heal.

I know this will be difficult to read, but you also need to break up with sugar. As we have already discussed, PCOS is associated with insulin resistance, which, because of its association with higher blood glucose levels, can lead to diabetes. Stop the progression in its tracks now. I am not instructing you to avoid all sugars or switch to artificial sweeteners. Focus on eating more natural, whole foods. These foods are typically higher in fiber, vitamins, and minerals, and they not only contribute to more stable blood sugar levels but can also fill you up so you are less likely to overeat.

Another goal should be to eliminate as many processed foods as possible from your diet. Processed foods often contain poor-quality fat and salt that can have a damaging effect on your body. If the food comes in a package and you don't recognize all the ingredients on the label, it is a processed food. Say goodbye.

I saved the most important habit to kick for last: You need to get rid of the mentality that eating special foods will "fix" your PCOS. I hate to be the bearer of bad news—there is no best diet for PCOS. I know you think you are reading a book about a specific diet, but what you are really reading is a book about a lifestyle. A lifestyle of eating whole, nutritious, delicious foods combined with regular activity and self-care all to help heal your PCOS.

EATING ADVICE

Although you should take into account what works best for you physically and emotionally, there are certain lifestyle practices that benefit women with PCOS, and I think they will help ensure your success.

One of the most important actions you can take to help control your PCOS symptoms is to have a plan when it comes to what you put into your body. Planning meals in advance helps you stay organized and in control of your food choices. You will know exactly what you are eating and when, and you can shop accordingly to have what you need to cook those healthy, delicious meals. No more random trips to the grocery store or orders of crave-indulging takeout. PCOS-healing meals are as close as your kitchen with this plan in place.

Most people live hectic lives and buying food for your next meal should not be a stressor. When you plan your food for both at-home meals and on-the-go snacks, you remove any uncertainty and stress. This preparedness also means you minimize the need to rely on fast food or waste money on unnecessary food items like munchies, sweets, and other treats that are not conducive to helping heal your PCOS. Remember, you are working toward removing all processed foods from your diet!

But what happens to your eating plan when things like holidays, special occasions, and restaurant events occur? Absolutely nothing. You have already planned for it. You can scan the menu ahead of time to select an item in tune with your goals, or you can call the host and ask what types of foods will be served. Once you know the potential challenges you'll face at the meal, you can come up with a game plan to ensure your success.

Another helpful practice to add to your success toolbox is to be mindful when you eat. Put down your phone or tablet and enjoy your food without electronics. Focus on the full ritual of eating: preparing the food, enjoying the enticing aromas, savoring the

A NIGHT ON THE TOWN

Right about now you might be feeling some apprehension about all these lifestyle changes. Maybe you're thinking that unless you stick to your diet and plan out every morsel you put in your mouth you will not be successful. That is SO far from the truth. In fact, every now and then we all deserve a night or day off from our diets.

I like to refer to these breaks as "reward meals." You are taking a conscious and intentional break from your normal healthy eating patterns. You are, therefore, rewarding good behavior.

If you have PCOS you are no stranger to food cravings. Constantly trying to resist your cravings can be exhausting. By indulging in a reward meal, you're able to relax because you have given yourself permission to indulge in your cravings.

Another benefit of reward meals is that many people are often able to resist temptation knowing there is light at the end of the tunnel. So, by allowing yourself to indulge in foods you generally don't eat, you may actually be more motivated to stay on track.

You may be scared of derailing and undoing all your hard work, but don't be. If you are intentional with your reward meals and have a plan, you will always be in control. Planning when and where your reward meal will occur is a great place to start. I suggest including a reward meal every two to three weeks. As you get closer to your goal weight, you can include a reward meal weekly. Continue to be mindful of your choices and enjoy the treat. You worked hard to earn it.

tastes and textures, recognizing when you're full, and participating in the community you bring together around your table. As you become more mindful, you can experiment with different amounts and combinations of foods. You'll also find that responding to true hunger—rather than eating out of boredom or stress—is one way to put the pleasure back in eating.

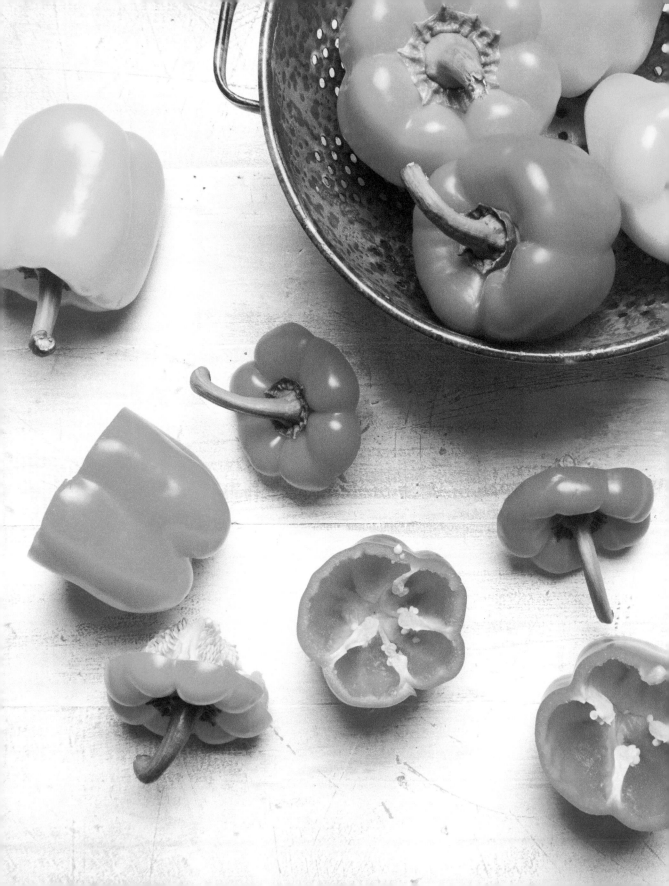

3.
THE DASH DIET

The Dietary Approaches to Stop Hypertension (DASH) diet—with a couple of little tweaks—is a perfect fit for women with PCOS. I have created a special version that stays true to the important health-enhancing principles of the traditional DASH diet while minimizing the overall carbohydrate content. The Modified DASH Diet for PCOS can promote weight loss, restore hormonal balance, and optimize insulin levels, all while decreasing a woman's risks of chronic disease.

DASH BASICS

According to the Centers for Disease Control, hypertension, or high blood pressure, is a serious health concern affecting more than 75 million Americans. High blood pressure, often referred to as the silent killer, frequently causes no visible symptoms and can go undetected for years. Fortunately, in 1990, researchers discovered two important things: Diet alone, without any medication, could effectively lower blood pressure, and certain nutrients appear to play an important role in this effect. Hence, the DASH diet was born.

A 2011 study published in *Current Hypertension Reports* established that what began as a dietary approach to reduce hypertension has become a well-revered and reliable plan for weight loss, diabetes prevention, insulin resistance, and cardiovascular disease. In fact, *U.S. News & World Report* ranked the DASH diet as the second "best overall" diet, comparing it against 40 other diets.

Even though the DASH diet wasn't originally designed for weight loss, it's no secret that many of the dietary factors that control blood pressure also influence weight. According to one study published in *Obesity Reviews*, adults who followed the DASH diet lost more weight in 8 to 24 weeks than those who adhered to other low-calorie diets. So, that might get you wondering, is there something magical that causes people to lose weight when following the DASH diet? Nope. The DASH diet just promotes a high-quality food plan rooted in portion control. It encourages eating low-calorie nutrient-dense food, lean sources of protein, and heart-healthy fat. It also discourages indulging in processed foods, poor-quality fat, and excess sugar.

The DASH diet not only decreases hypertension, but research supports that the diet can be highly effective in managing insulin resistance. As with weight loss, these positive benefits are attributed to the actual composition of the DASH diet, as well as the emphasis on portion control. Additionally, in 2004, in the PREMIER trial, 54 participants were randomly assigned to one of three dietary interventions for hypertension. Based on the results, the authors concluded that eating foods recommended by the DASH diet, in conjunction with a very low-calorie diet, could lead to significant improvements in insulin sensitivity.

The DASH diet is a tool anyone can use to create a healthy lifestyle. Followers of this diet can take comfort in the fact that their food choices are endorsed not only by extensive research, but also by some of the most respected medical organizations in the world, including the National Institutes of Health, the Academy of Nutrition and Dietetics, and the American Heart Association.

DASH DIET GUIDELINES

The DASH diet doesn't rely on specific foods, but instead provides recommendations for specific servings of seven main food groups: vegetables; fruits; whole grains; low-fat dairy; lean proteins; nuts, seeds, and legumes; and healthy fat. The number of servings allowed is relative to your total calorie intake. Therefore, the more calories your body needs the more servings per food group you can eat. Note that although the DASH diet recommends certain foods, many foods are also discouraged, including processed foods, fried foods, excess sweets, high amounts of alcohol, and excessive salt. The good news is that the DASH diet supports eating all of the following:

Vegetables. The DASH diet highly favors vegetables—and with good reason. Vegetables are high in fiber, potassium, and antioxidants. All vegetables are allowed on the DASH diet. Because each vegetable supplies different nutrients, variety is encouraged.

Fruits. If you follow the traditional DASH approach, you'll see there is a strong emphasis on fruit. Although fruit is a wonderful source of potassium, antioxidants, and fiber, it also contains sugar. Therefore, when I explain the specific dietary guidelines for women with PCOS, you will see some slight changes in the recommendations for fruit. Like vegetables, all fruits are allowed on the DASH diet and variety is encouraged to maximize your intake of the various nutrients.

Whole Grains. Whole grains are full of fiber, magnesium, and potassium that support virtually every system in the body. The fiber in whole grains is digested slowly, releasing sugar and insulin at a stable rate that helps with feeling full. Whole grains include products with the word "whole" listed as the first ingredient—such as in whole-grain breads and wraps and whole-grain breakfast cereals—brown rice, bulgur, quinoa, and oatmeal.

Dairy Products. Dairy products on the DASH diet are recommended to be low in fat. Full-fat dairy is high in saturated fat and is not considered heart-healthy. Dairy products are great sources of calcium, vitamin D, and magnesium that support bone and cardiovascular health. Examples of low-fat dairy include skim milk, low-fat cheese, and low-fat yogurt.

Poultry, Meat, and Fish. On the DASH diet you will be getting your protein from a variety of sources. The DASH diet encourages eggs and lean cuts of meat, fish, and poultry. Although the DASH diet hasn't been specifically tested in vegetarians, it can be easily adapted by including plant-based protein sources such as soy, legumes, low-fat dairy, and beans. Red meat intake is limited to no more than one or two servings per week.

Nuts, Seeds, and Legumes. Nuts, seeds, and legumes are excellent sources of magnesium, fiber, and heart-healthy fat. Legumes include lentils, kidney beans, navy beans, black beans, peanuts, chickpeas, split peas, and soybeans. Although nuts are healthy, be mindful that a small amount provides a concentrated source of calories, so consume them just a couple of times per week, or in small quantities.

Heart-Healthy Fat. Heart-healthy fat—such as avocado, nuts and seeds, and extra-virgin olive oil—is an integral part of the DASH diet. Fat helps keep us feeling full and provides flavor and nutrients with many important cardiovascular benefits.

THREE STEPS TO KICK-START YOUR DASH DIET

1. **Mind-set and motivation.** Mind-set is everything. It is critical that before you start the DASH diet you make sure you are in the right mind-set. A good way to ensure this is to establish clear reasons for embarking on this journey. By establishing a clear "why," you will be able to rise above any temptations or obstacles that may surface. You might want to solidify your motivations further by writing them down and keeping them visible. If urges for unhealthy food arise, you can always reread your list of motivations to reinforce your commitment.

2. **A no-diet approach.** Although "diet" is inherent in its name, the DASH diet is by no means a traditional diet in the sense that it does not rely on restriction for results. The DASH diet is based on eating nutrient-dense foods, appropriately portioned, that are nourishing and provide a high level of satiety. Although this will enhance weight loss, you will never feel deprived. In addition, the DASH diet is not something you stop doing once you have reached your goals. It is an eating pattern that is sustainable and can be followed indefinitely. Developing a no-diet approach is critical to your success.

3. **Bulletproof your life.** Changing eating patterns can be difficult no matter how flexible or accommodating the new pattern may be. Begin by bulletproofing your environment: Clear cupboards, cabinets, and your refrigerator of any foods that might encourage unhealthy eating patterns. Prep any food you can ahead of time to enhance your dedication and compliance. Divide larger bags of calorie-dense foods, like nuts and seeds, into smaller bags to decrease the desire to over-consume portions. Do whatever it takes to ensure success.

PCOS AND THE DASH DIET

Though originally created for managing high blood pressure, the DASH diet can also be extremely beneficial for women suffering from PCOS—women who are at an increased risk of chronic diseases such as heart disease, diabetes, and obesity. In addition, studies show these women often experience insulin resistance and higher levels of inflammation than the general population. Therefore, dietary strategies for women with PCOS must address these health consequences to be considered an effective treatment strategy. So, let's take a deeper look at exactly how the DASH diet can help alleviate the incidence of these diseases, as well as enhance the lifestyle of women with PCOS.

HOW DOES THE DASH DIET WORK FOR WOMEN WITH PCOS?

Diet and lifestyle modifications are, without question, the most important strategies for improving PCOS symptoms. But as we have discussed, the symptoms are complex. For a lifestyle change to be effective, it must address the underlying metabolic and hormonal disruptions of the disease. The DASH diet does just that. The DASH diet is a near-perfect fit for women with PCOS. At its core, the DASH diet helps minimize insulin resistance and can lead to major improvements in the overall health of women with PCOS. When followed properly, the diet can promote weight loss, restore hormonal balance, and optimize insulin levels, all while decreasing a woman's risks of chronic disease. Let's examine why the DASH diet works so well for women with PCOS.

Optimized Insulin Levels. Reducing insulin levels and improving insulin sensitivity are paramount in the management of PCOS. Therefore, it comes as no surprise that both the quality and quantity of carbohydrates consumed are critical. The DASH diet emphasizes whole grains and appropriate serving sizes for women with PCOS. Because of their fiber content, whole grains minimize spikes in blood sugar and insulin levels because they are digested more slowly. Individuals who are insulin sensitive are better able to manage their weight and experience a reduced risk of diabetes, heart disease, and obesity when they consume whole grains. Lower levels of insulin are also consistent with menstrual regularity, which further facilitates a decrease in the symptoms of PCOS.

Rock-Star Nutrients. Fruits and vegetables are the cornerstones of the DASH diet, making the diet naturally high in nutrients such as calcium, potassium, magnesium, and antioxidants. Collectively these nutrients hold rock-star status in the body. They serve many important roles—from regulating blood pressure to minimizing inflammation. Research indicates that women with PCOS are more likely to experience higher inflammatory markers in the body. This increase in chronic inflammation in PCOS is concerning as it increases the risk of cardiovascular disease, as well as fertility problems. But by following a lower-inflammatory diet, women with PCOS can experience a decrease in their overall symptoms and significantly reduce their likelihood of developing a chronic disease like heart disease or diabetes.

More Fiber. Please! The DASH diet is chock-full of fiber. The Dietary Guidelines for Americans recommend that women consume at least 25 grams of fiber per day. Thanks to the DASH diet's reliance on fresh fruits, veggies, whole grains, nuts, and seeds, achieving this goal is no problem. As already noted, women with PCOS are more likely to develop diabetes, insulin resistance, high cholesterol, and obesity. Consuming sufficient fiber can help effectively manage these conditions. Foods that contain fiber enter the bloodstream more slowly than other foods. In response, the body releases blood sugar more slowly and at a more even rate. This reaction minimizes surges in blood sugar and insulin and helps prevent the progression of diabetes and insulin resistance. In addition, when blood sugar and insulin levels are stable, cravings are minimized. Diets that are high in fiber are also effective in controlling cholesterol. Fiber binds the excess cholesterol circulating in the body so the body can dispose of it in stool, thereby lowering overall cholesterol levels. Finally, fiber expands in the stomach and promotes a feeling of fullness, which can prevent overeating and excess weight gain.

DIETARY GUIDELINES

The Modified DASH Diet for PCOS doesn't require you to count calories. Yay! It delivers high-quality foods full of important nutrients that work with your PCOS, not against it. But why *modified*? One thing that has stood out as I've worked with women with PCOS is that most do not process carbohydrates well. That is not to say they can't have any; rather, they need to be cautious about carbohydrate serving sizes. So, although the majority of carbohydrates on the traditional DASH plan are complex, I have made a few modifications to enhance the dietary goals of women with PCOS.

I recognize not every woman suffering from PCOS desires weight loss. Therefore, I have created two different sets of guidelines: one for women who want to lose weight and one for women content with their weight and who seek weight maintenance. Please be mindful that these serve as basic guidelines for your daily eating patterns. The goal is to meet these recommendations *most* days. So don't sweat the small things if meeting the goal doesn't happen every day.

DIETARY GUIDELINES FOR THE MODIFIED DASH DIET FOR PCOS

	SERVING SIZE	WEIGHT LOSS SERVINGS	WEIGHT MAINTENANCE SERVINGS
Non-starchy Vegetables	One serving equals: 1 cup of raw, leafy green vegetables; ½ cup sliced vegetables, raw or cooked, such as cucumbers, green beans, and peppers	Unlimited, minimum of 3 per day	Unlimited, minimum of 4 per day
*Fruits	One serving equals: 1 medium whole fruit; ½ cup fresh, frozen, or canned fruit; ¼ cup dried fruit	2 per day	3 per day
*Whole Grains and Starchy Vegetables	One serving equals: ½ cup cooked brown rice, whole-grain or whole-wheat pasta, or whole-grain cereal; 1 slice whole-grain bread; 1 ounce dry whole-grain cereal; ½ cup cooked peas or corn; ¾ cup cooked winter squash; ⅓ cup cooked sweet potato	3 or 4 per day	5 or 6 per day
Dairy	One serving equals: 1 cup low-fat milk (skim or 1 percent); 1 cup low-fat yogurt; ½ cup low-fat ricotta; ½ cup low-sodium, low-fat cottage cheese; 1½ ounces low-fat cheese	2 or 3 per day	2 or 3 per day
Nuts, Seeds, Beans and Legumes	One serving equals: ⅓ cup nuts; 2 tablespoons peanut butter; 2 tablespoons seeds	3 or 4 per week	3 or 4 per week
Lean Meat, Fish, Poultry, and Eggs	One serving equals: 3 ounces cooked lean meat, skinless poultry, or fish; 1 large egg; 2 large egg whites	2 or 3 per day	2 or 3 per day
Heart-Healthy Fat	One serving equals: 1 teaspoon soft margarine, vegetable oil, canola oil, or extra-virgin olive oil; 1 tablespoon olive oil–based mayonnaise; 2 tablespoons low-fat salad dressing or 1 tablespoon regular dressing	3 or 4 per day	3 or 4 per day

*The serving sizes suggested for fruit, whole grains, and starchy vegetables have been modified from the original DASH program in an effort to decrease the overall total carbohydrate content for women with PCOS.

As you can see, there is no shortage of delicious foods to choose from. The following section discusses in detail the various food groups you can enjoy while following the Modified DASH Diet for PCOS.

Non-starchy vegetables. Vegetables are low in calories and loaded with vitamins, minerals, fiber, and disease-fighting antioxidants. They are a fantastic way to fill up! Examples include foods such as asparagus, broccoli, Brussels sprouts, cabbage, cauliflower, cucumbers, eggplant, lettuce, peppers, tomatoes, and yellow and green squash. There are no limits on the amounts of non-starchy vegetables you can consume.

Fruit. Fruit is high in nutrients and fiber, and can be a quick and convenient snack, but it is also a source of carbohydrates. Including fruit, especially berries, in your diet is encouraged, but be mindful of the quantity. Excessive amounts of fruit consumed in one sitting can spike sugar and insulin levels that, in turn, can affect weight. So, please don't shy away from fruit, just do your best to stick to the suggested quantities.

Whole grains and starchy vegetables. Diets high in carbohydrates can be detrimental for women who have PCOS; evidence, however, doesn't support the benefits of significantly reducing your intake of them either. Therefore, moderate amounts of whole grains are encouraged on the Modified DASH Diet for PCOS. Examples of whole grains include amaranth, barley, brown rice, buckwheat, bulgur, quinoa, whole oats, and whole-wheat bread. When purchasing bread always look for the words "whole wheat" or "whole grain" listed as the first ingredient. We include the starchy vegetables—corn, peas, sweet potatoes, and winter squashes (acorn and butternut)—in this category because they are relatively higher in carbohydrates than non-starchy vegetables.

Dairy products. Low-fat dairy products are important for women with PCOS. They are great sources of calcium, vitamin D, and protein. Studies have documented that sufficient calcium can help lower your blood pressure, strengthen your bones and even aid in weight loss. Examples include low-fat milk (skim or 1 percent), low-fat yogurt, low-fat ricotta, low-sodium and low-fat cottage cheese, and low-fat cheeses like Cheddar, mozzarella, Parmigiano-Reggiano, and Swiss.

Poultry, meat, fish, eggs, beans, and legumes. Protein is critical for women with PCOS. Consuming sufficient amounts of protein with meals and snacks can increase satiety and decrease hunger between meals. The goal is to choose lean sources of protein, such as eggs and egg whites, fish, seafood, and skinless poultry. Red meat can be enjoyed in moderation, limiting it to one or two servings per week. Try to choose leaner cuts of meat, which include round, sirloin, flank, tenderloin, and ground round. Beans and legumes are included in this group because of their relatively high amounts of protein. They are nutrition powerhouses, but they also contain carbohydrates. Therefore, unless you exclusively follow a plant-based diet, I recommend diversifying your protein with the majority coming from poultry, eggs, and fish.

Nuts and seeds. Nuts (such as black beans, chickpeas, kidney beans, lentils, navy beans, peanuts, split peas, and soybeans) and seeds (chia, pumpkin, and sunflower) make a great snack for women with PCOS. They are high in fiber and contain a modest amount of protein, keeping us satisfied and full. Despite the fact that nuts are very healthy, we need to pay careful attention to our allotted portion sizes and servings per week, as they do provide a concentrated amount of calories.

Heart-healthy fat. Heart-healthy fat is vital for women with PCOS, including mono-unsaturated fat and polyunsaturated fat, such as avocado, canola oil, extra-virgin olive oil, and vegetable oil. These kinds of fat are considered heart-healthy because they help improve our cholesterol levels and ward off cardiovascular disease. Although these types of fat are more helpful than others, all fat contains about the same amount of calories. So, when it comes to fat, consider both the type and amount.

FOODS TO AVOID

The great part about the Modified DASH Diet for PCOS is that there are so many healthy and delicious foods allowed, which means the list of foods to avoid is rather short. Whereas nothing is totally off limits, certain foods are discouraged, including:

- Processed meats
- Red meat in excessive amounts
- Sugary beverages
- Sweets

Also, not all fat is created equal. Saturated fat and trans fat both can have adverse impacts on our cholesterol levels and overall health. Saturated fat is found in red meats; full-fat dairy products such as cheese, milk, and butter; and the skin of poultry. Trans fat, or hydrogenated fat, is found in processed foods—cakes, pastries, cookies, potato chips, and fried foods.

If you are wondering whether your cup of joe in the morning or your nightly glass of Merlot is off limits, you'll be happy to know there is room for these indulgences—within reason. The Modified DASH Diet for PCOS does not limit nor endorse caffeine, as research on its impact on hypertension and overall health appears inconclusive. In some populations, studies have shown that alcohol has demonstrated the ability to raise blood pressure. Therefore, although not completely off limits, women are encouraged to consume one or fewer drinks daily.

DASH PREP

Here you will discover how to best prepare yourself to adopt the Modified DASH Diet for PCOS. Getting yourself organized is critical to ensuring success. As you will see, I have done my best to ease you into this way of eating by providing some basic tips and guidelines to get started.

I offer information on the refrigerator and pantry staples I feel are most helpful to have on hand. Remember, the goal of all of this is to establish healthy eating patterns you can sustain for the rest of your life. If there are ingredients or foods on this list that you have tried and don't like, just omit them. Keep in mind there is very little actual restriction on food choices, so please just choose the ones you really enjoy—keeping an open mind to try new foods when you feel ready.

Having the right ingredients and foods to whip up healthy and delicious meals is only half the equation, though. You also need to have the right equipment. You may already have many of the kitchen items described in the essential equipment section (see page 41), but keep in mind I created this list for the beginner cook. I have done my best to include only those items I consider truly essential. I am a big believer that having the proper equipment can make a huge difference in your results in the kitchen. However, you don't need to break the bank. All the items described can be easily purchased at either your favorite retail or discount store. Even better, you can check out yard sales or your local Salvation Army or Goodwill store to score some great buys on kitchen equipment.

Finally, I include helpful tips and guidelines on how to make your transition to the Modified DASH Diet for PCOS as easy as possible. Although you may find some of these suggestions common knowledge, rigorously adhering to them will help you avoid any potential roadblocks and stay on track. Embarking on a new way of eating can be hard. But staying organized and taking the time to prepare will improve your odds of sticking with this plan that can ultimately alleviate many of your PCOS symptoms.

REFRIGERATOR AND PANTRY ITEMS

The foods and ingredients you choose to keep in your kitchen should be dictated by your personal taste and preferences. I know this may sound straightforward, but you should only eat foods you enjoy. I am not saying don't try new foods. In fact, I encourage variety in all areas of your diet. But I don't want you to force yourself to eat something you don't like just because it is healthy. Remember, this is a lifestyle, not a diet. Here are some suggestions for items to put in your grocery cart to get you started.

Foods High in Protein and Low in Saturated Fat

- Cheeses, low-fat, such as Cheddar, mozzarella, Parmigiano-Reggiano, Swiss

- Eggs, organic

- Fish, all types, such as cod, salmon, sole, tuna

- Meats, lean, such as skinless chicken breasts and pork tenderloin

- Yogurt, low-fat plain Greek

Heart-Healthy Fat

- Avocado

- Nuts, such as almonds, pecans, walnuts; and seeds, such as sunflower seeds

- Oils, such as canola, extra-virgin olive, nut, vegetable

Whole Grains

- Brown rice, bulgur, old-fashioned oats, quinoa, whole-grain bread, wild rice

The Rest of Your Cart

- All vegetables, including broccoli; cucumbers; eggplant; lettuces, such as arugula, Boston Bibb, and spring mix; scallions, tomatoes—whatever looks good and is in season

- Dried herbs, such as chili powder, cumin, curry powder, ginger, and herbes de Provence

- Fresh fruit, such as blueberries, raspberries, and strawberries

- Fresh herbs and spices, such as basil, cilantro, garlic, mint, and thyme

- Vinegars, such as apple cider, balsamic, red wine, rice

ESSENTIAL EQUIPMENT

This equipment list is geared toward the beginner cook for daily cooking. This list is by no means all-inclusive, but does provide you with the basic equipment to get started in the kitchen.

Baking sheets and sheet pans: These are perfect for roasting vegetables and baking poultry and fish.

Chef's knife: Get a good quality 8-inch knife; your new way of eating is going to include a lot of chopping. A comfortable, sharp knife will be one of your most important tools.

Colander: A metal or ceramic colander can be used for draining pasta and beans, as well as for washing fruits and vegetables.

Cutting board: A sturdy cutting board is a must for any cook.

Glass baking dishes: You should have 8-by-8-inch and 9-by-13-inch sizes; glass pans are good heat insulators, easy to clean, and don't warp like metal pans can.

Grill pan: Get the delicious taste of grilled foods without leaving the comfort of your kitchen.

Instant-read thermometer: This is a must for judging correct doneness temperatures when cooking poultry and meat.

Large stockpot: You'll need this for making soups, big batches of sauce, and boiling water for pasta and potatoes.

Measuring cups and measuring spoons: Measuring your food ensures accuracy and helps you achieve the desired results.

Mixing bowls: It's best to have small, medium, and large sizes for various uses, including mixing dry ingredients, holding chopped vegetables, and mixing sauces.

Nonstick skillets: The 8-inch and 10-inch sizes are great for cooking just about everything, and nonstick means you don't need to add much oil.

THIS BOOK'S RECIPES

The recipes in this book include the following labels, when applicable, to help you best meet your needs on any particular day:

5-Ingredient: uses only 5 main ingredients or fewer

30-Minute: can be made in 30 minutes or less—start to finish

Fertility Booster: contains a full serving of either heart-healthy fat, whole grains, vegetables, and/or fish or plant-based protein

Inflammation Fighter: includes ingredients that help fight inflammation

Lower Calorie: contains 200 or fewer calories per serving to assist with weight loss

All of the recipes include easy-to-find ingredients and are based on foods that are beneficial in healing PCOS symptoms. The directions are simple and straightforward, allowing even the novice cook to flourish in the kitchen. So grab your apron, and let's get cooking!

TIPS FOR SUCCESS

Establishing new habits can be hard. Here are six tips to help you ease into your new eating patterns.

1. Schedule specific days and times directly into your calendar during which you will plan, shop, and meal prep. By allocating the necessary time, you can avoid the excuse, "I don't have time to cook and eat healthfully."

2. Use grocery stores that allow you to order food online and have it either delivered to your home or available for pick-up already bagged to go. Of course, these services cost extra, but they can save you time and money in the long run.

3. Sometimes salad bars can be your best friend for scooping up precut vegetables, hardboiled eggs, and, if you are lucky, precooked grilled chicken. Although more expensive than purchasing the items whole or uncooked, they are convenient in a pinch when you are short on time and energy.

4. Whenever possible, use single servings of foods like yogurts, cheese sticks, nuts, and seeds. These little lifesavers cut down on prep time and help you stay on track—especially when snacking.

5. If your grocery store has them, bulk bins are a great way to add variety into your diet without breaking the bank. Bulk bins offer a wide variety of whole grains, nuts, seeds, and dried fruit at a much lower price than packaged options.

6. Wash and prep fruits and vegetables before putting them away. Though it may be the last thing you want to do after lugging in your bounty, you will be so happy to have clean and already-sliced red pepper, cucumber, and celery ready to munch on when the urge hits for a snack.

CURB YOUR CRAVINGS

Everyone experiences food cravings, but women with PCOS are more susceptible to them. The culprit for the intense cravings? High insulin levels.

Insulin is an appetite stimulant that can create strong cravings—especially for sweets. The more sweets you eat, the more you crave. Whereas the Modified DASH Diet for PCOS will certainly help minimize these cravings, use these quick tips to reduce their temptation further.

Limit high-sugar foods. High-sugar foods such as baked goods, bagels, candy, and sweet drinks all contribute to cravings. They cause blood sugar and insulin levels to rise quickly, which then plummet shortly thereafter. When sugar levels drop, the vicious cycle starts again.

Pump up the protein. If you find yourself craving sugar, it could be related to your protein intake. Getting sufficient protein with your meals and snacks can stabilize your blood sugar and help you feel full and satisfied between meals. Plus, protein has little effect on insulin levels.

Move it, sister. Stress can be a contributing factor for cravings, and we have already learned that women with PCOS have no shortage of stress. Make sure you include regular exercise in your daily routine to combat stress and reduce cravings. Also, don't forget to incorporate mindfulness activities, like yoga, meditation, and deep breathing, which also reduce stress.

MEAL PLANS

In the pages that follow I have provided three weeks of meal plans to jump-start your weight loss on the Modified DASH Diet for PCOS. **NOTE:** If you are currently at your goal weight, please add one to two servings of fruits and one to two servings of whole grains and/or starchy vegetables to what is suggested in the daily meal plans.

 If you follow a vegetarian diet, I have included alternatives where necessary. However, please be aware that the additional beans and whole grains will result in a higher carbohydrate intake. This doesn't mean you won't lose weight while following this plan; it just means the weight loss might be slower.

WEEK ONE

Day 1

BREAKFAST

Mushroom and Asparagus Quinoa Frittata (page 66) with 1 cup of strawberries

LUNCH

Vegetable and White Bean Soup (page 82)

DINNER

Chili-Lime Chicken Fajitas with Mango Salsa (page 104)

Vegetarian Alternative: Creamy Lentils with Kale, Spinach, and Artichoke Hearts (page 89)

SNACK

Balsamic Berries and Ricotta (page 129)

Tip: Add 1 low-fat cheese stick to balance out your day.

Day 2

◔ BREAKFAST

Superfood Green Smoothie (page 69)

● LUNCH

Leftovers: Chili-Lime Chicken Fajitas with Mango Salsa (page 104)

Vegetarian Alternative: Leftovers: Creamy Lentils with Kale, Spinach, and Artichoke Hearts (page 89)

◒ DINNER

Quinoa and Black Bean Bowls with Cilantro Vinaigrette (page 76)

○ SNACK

Oatmeal Dark Chocolate Chip Peanut Butter Cookies (page 130)

Tip: Add 8 ounces low-fat milk to balance out your day.

Day 3

◔ BREAKFAST

Spicy Baked Eggs with Goat Cheese and Spinach (page 64) with small orange

● LUNCH

Leftovers: Quinoa and Black Bean Bowls with Cilantro Vinaigrette (page 76)

◒ DINNER

Pistachio-Encrusted Salmon (page 107) with Roasted Vegetables (page 126)

Vegetarian Alternative: Vegetable Moo Shu Wraps (page 94)

○ SNACK

Leftovers: Oatmeal Dark Chocolate Chip Peanut Butter Cookies (page 130)

Tip: Add 8 ounces low-fat milk to balance out your day.

Day 4

◔ BREAKFAST

Overnight Apple and Chia Seed Refrigerator Oatmeal (page 65)

● LUNCH

Leftovers: Pistachio-Encrusted Salmon (page 107) with Roasted Vegetables (page 126)

Vegetarian Alternative: Leftovers: Vegetable Moo Shu Wraps (page 94)

◡ DINNER

French Lentil Salad (page 78)

○ SNACK

Honey-Roasted Sunflower and Pumpkin Seeds (page 128)

Tip: Add 8 ounces low-fat plain or Greek yogurt to balance out your day.

Day 5

◔ BREAKFAST

Ricotta Toast with Tomato and Cucumber (page 68) with 1 cup blackberries

● LUNCH

Leftovers: French Lentil Salad (page 78)

◡ DINNER

Hearty Chili (page 80) with Green Beans with Toasted Almonds (page 127)

○ SNACK

Leftovers: Honey-Roasted Sunflower and Pumpkin Seeds (page 128)

Tip: Add 8 ounces low-fat plain Greek yogurt to balance out your day.

Day 6

⌒ BREAKFAST

Mushroom and Asparagus Quinoa Frittata (page 66) with small banana

● LUNCH

Vegetable and Hummus Pita (page 83)

⌣ DINNER

Leftovers: Hearty Chili (page 80) with Green Beans with Toasted Almonds (page 127)

○ SNACK

Roasted Vegetables (page 126)

Tip: Add 1½ ounces low-fat cheese to balance out your day.

Day 7

⌒ BREAKFAST

Whole-Grain Flax Waffles with Strawberry Purée (page 62)

● LUNCH

Vegetable and White Bean Soup (page 82)

⌣ DINNER

Artichoke Chicken (page 103) with steamed carrots and 1 teaspoon butter

Vegetarian Alternative: Vegetarian Spaghetti Squash Casserole (page 95)

○ SNACK

Balsamic Berries and Ricotta (page 129)

Tip: Add 8 ounces low-fat milk to balance out your day.

Day 1

◔ BREAKFAST

Spicy Baked Eggs with Goat Cheese and Spinach (page 64) with 1 cup grapes

● LUNCH

Fennel-Apple-Walnut Salad (page 75)

◓ DINNER

Pasta Primavera (page 90) with a side salad tossed with 2 teaspoons Balsamic Vinaigrette (page 135)

○ SNACK

Green Beans with Toasted Almonds (page 127)

Tip: Add ½ cup low-sodium, low-fat cottage cheese to balance out your day.

Day 2

◔ BREAKFAST

Superfood Green Smoothie (page 69)

● LUNCH

Vegetarian Stuffed Peppers (page 88)

◓ DINNER

Leftovers: Pasta Primavera (page 90) with a side salad tossed with 2 teaspoons Balsamic Vinaigrette (page 135)

○ SNACK

Balsamic Berries and Ricotta (page 129)

Tip: Add ⅓ cup nuts to balance out your day.

Day 3

◖ BREAKFAST

Pineapple-Banana High-Protein Smoothie (page 70)

● LUNCH

Sweet Potato and Black Bean Tortillas with Avocado Yogurt Sauce (page 86)

◗ DINNER

Leftovers: Vegetarian Stuffed Peppers (page 88)

○ SNACK

Leftovers: Balsamic Berries and Ricotta (page 129)

Tip: Add 1½ ounces low-fat cheese to balance out your day.

Day 4

◖ BREAKFAST

Overnight Apple and Chia Seed Refrigerator Oatmeal (page 65)

● LUNCH

Shrimp Noodle Bowls with Ginger Broth (page 108)

Vegetarian Alternative: Creamy Lentils with Kale, Spinach, and Artichoke Hearts (page 89)

◗ DINNER

Leftovers: Sweet Potato and Black Bean Tortillas with Avocado Yogurt Sauce (page 86)

○ SNACK

Portobello Mushrooms with Ricotta, Tomato, and Mozzarella (page 124)

Day 5

◖ BREAKFAST

Mushroom and Asparagus Quinoa Frittata (page 66) with 2 clementines

● LUNCH

Leftovers: Shrimp Noodle Bowls with Ginger Broth (page 108)

Vegetarian Alternative: Leftovers: Creamy Lentils with Kale, Spinach, and Artichoke Hearts (page 89)

◗ DINNER

Apricot Chicken (page 102)

Vegetarian Alternative: Vegetable Moo Shu Wraps (page 94)

○ SNACK

Pinto Bean–Stuffed Sweet Potatoes (page 125)

Tip: Add 8 ounces low-fat milk to balance out your day.

Day 6

◖ BREAKFAST

Ricotta Toast with Tomato and Cucumber (page 68) with 1 small plum

● LUNCH

Leftovers: Apricot Chicken (page 102)

Vegetarian Alternative: Leftovers: Vegetable Moo Shu Wraps (page 94)

◗ DINNER

Roasted Tomato and Barley Risotto (page 92) with a side salad tossed with 2 teaspoons Balsamic Vinaigrette (page 135)

SNACK

Roasted Vegetables (page 126)

Tip: Add 2 tablespoons sunflower seeds to balance out your day.

Day 7

BREAKFAST

Superfood Green Smoothie (page 69)

LUNCH

Leftovers: Roasted Tomato and Barley Risotto (page 92) with a side salad tossed with 2 teaspoons Balsamic Vinaigrette (page 135)

DINNER

Italian Beef Stew (page 115)

Vegetarian Alternative: Pinto Bean–Stuffed Sweet Potatoes (page 125) with Roasted Vegetables (page 126)

SNACK

Green Beans with Toasted Almonds (page 127)

Tip: Add 8 ounces low-fat plain or Greek yogurt to balance out your day.

WEEK THREE

Day 1

BREAKFAST

Pineapple-Banana High-Protein Smoothie (page 70)

LUNCH

Thai Pork in Lettuce Cups (page 117)

Vegetarian Alternative: Hearty Chili (page 80), excluding the ground beef

DINNER

Leftovers: Italian Beef Stew (page 115)

Vegetarian Alternative: Pinto Bean–Stuffed Sweet Potatoes (page 125) with Roasted Vegetables (page 126)

SNACK

Honey-Roasted Sunflower and Pumpkin Seeds (page 128)

Tip: Add 8 ounces low-fat milk to balance out your day.

Day 2

BREAKFAST

Spicy Baked Eggs with Goat Cheese and Spinach (page 64) with 1 small pear

LUNCH

Leftovers: Thai Pork in Lettuce Cups (page 117)

Vegetarian Alternative: Leftovers: Hearty Chili (page 80), excluding the ground beef

DINNER

Grilled Flank Steak with Peach Compote (page 114) served with ½ cup cooked quinoa and Green Beans with Toasted Almonds (page 127)

Vegetarian Alternative: French Lentil Salad (page 78) with Green Beans with Toasted Almonds (page 127)

SNACK

Balsamic Berries and Ricotta (page 129)

Tip: Add 1 cup raw veggies of your choice to balance out your day.

Day 3

BREAKFAST

Whole-Grain Flax Waffles with Strawberry Purée (page 62)

LUNCH

Leftovers: Grilled Flank Steak with Peach Compote (page 114) with a side salad tossed with 2 teaspoons Balsamic Vinaigrette (page 135)

Vegetarian Alternative: Leftovers: French Lentil Salad (page 78) with Green Beans with Toasted Almonds (page 127)

DINNER

Mushroom and Asparagus Quinoa Frittata (page 66) with steamed Brussels sprouts tossed with 2 teaspoons Simple Vinaigrette (page 134)

SNACK

Oatmeal Dark Chocolate Chip Peanut Butter Cookies (page 130)

Tip: Add 8 ounces low-fat milk to balance out your day.

Day 4

BREAKFAST

Overnight Apple and Chia Seed Refrigerator Oatmeal (page 65)

LUNCH

Leftovers: Mushroom and Asparagus Quinoa Frittata (page 66) with 1 cup raspberries

DINNER

Artichoke Chicken (page 103)

Vegetarian Alternative: Pasta Primavera (page 90)

SNACK

Leftovers: Oatmeal Dark Chocolate Chip Peanut Butter Cookies (page 130)

Tip: Add 8 ounces low-fat milk to balance out your day.

Day 5

BREAKFAST

Ricotta Toast with Tomato and Cucumber (page 68) with 1 small nectarine

LUNCH

Spaghetti Squash with Meat Sauce (page 112)

Vegetarian Alternative: Vegetarian Spaghetti Squash Casserole (page 95)

DINNER

Pinto Bean–Stuffed Sweet Potatoes (page 125)

SNACK

¼ cup Homemade Hummus (page 137) and 1 cup sliced red bell peppers

Day 6

BREAKFAST

Mushroom and Asparagus Quinoa Frittata (page 66) with 1 small peach

LUNCH

Three-Bean Vegetable Salad (page 74)

DINNER

Leftovers: Spaghetti Squash with Meat Sauce (page 112)

Vegetarian Alternative: Leftovers: Vegetarian Spaghetti Squash Casserole (page 95)

SNACK

Leftovers: Balsamic Berries and Ricotta (page 129)

Tip: Add ⅓ cup nuts to balance out your day.

Day 7

BREAKFAST

Pineapple-Banana High-Protein Smoothie (page 70)

LUNCH

Vegetable and Hummus Pita (page 83)

DINNER

Roasted Tomato and Barley Risotto (page 92)

SNACK

Portobello Mushrooms with Ricotta, Tomato, and Mozzarella (page 124)

Tip: Add ¼ cup Honey-Roasted Sunflower and Pumpkin Seeds (page 128) to balance out your day.

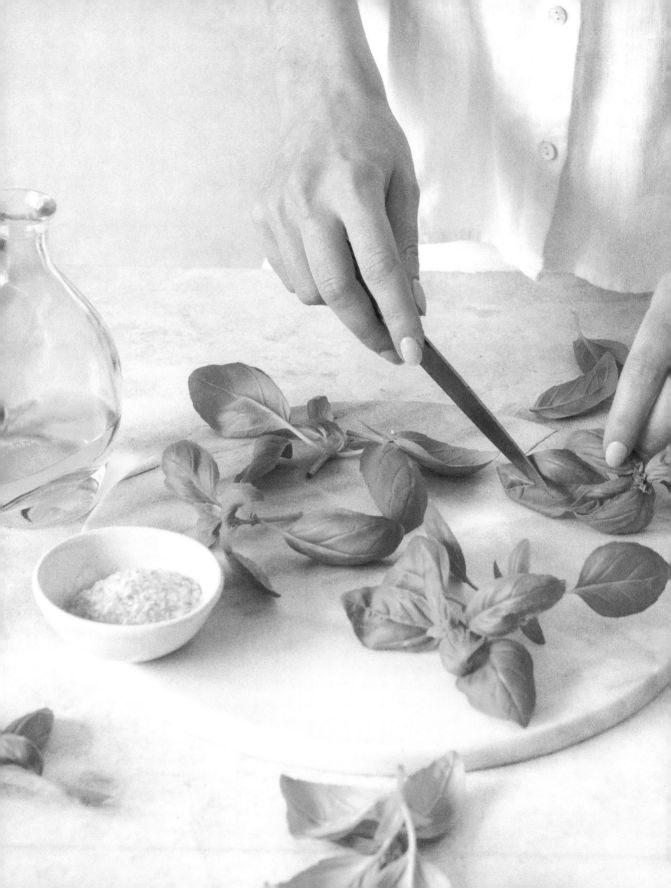

Part Two

THE RECIPES

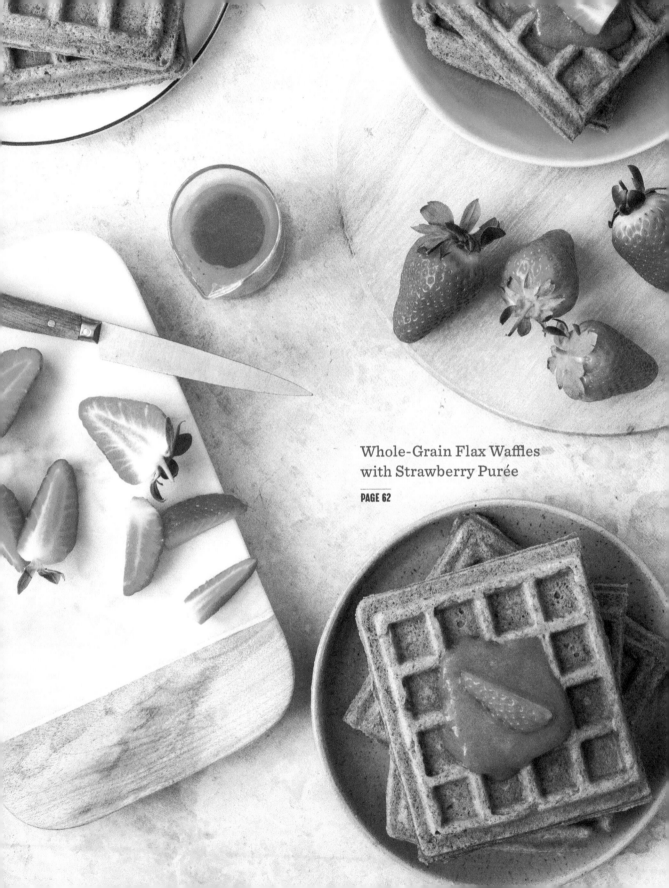

Whole-Grain Flax Waffles
with Strawberry Purée

PAGE 62

4.
BREAKFAST AND SMOOTHIES

WHOLE-GRAIN FLAX WAFFLES WITH STRAWBERRY PURÉE

30-Minute

Prep time: 15 minutes   **Cook time:** 15 minutes   **Total time:** 30 minutes

Waffles are known for being crispy on the outside and fluffy and tender on the inside—and this version is no exception. I've added a boost of nutrition with whole-wheat pastry flour and flaxseed, but the texture remains delicate and mouthwatering. The strawberry purée, a lower-sugar substitute for maple syrup, provides a tangy sweetness. *Serves 6*

FOR THE STRAWBERRY PURÉE
1 quart fresh strawberries, hulled and chopped

1 cup water

2 tablespoons honey

½ teaspoon vanilla extract

FOR THE WAFFLES
2¼ cups whole-wheat flour or whole-wheat pastry flour

¼ cup ground flaxseed

2½ teaspoons baking powder

1 teaspoon baking soda

½ teaspoon kosher salt

¼ cup canola oil

2 tablespoons dark brown sugar

2 teaspoons ground cinnamon

3 large eggs

2 teaspoons vanilla extract

1 cup nonfat milk

Nonstick cooking spray, for cooking the waffles

To make the strawberry purée

In a medium saucepan over medium heat, combine the strawberries, water, honey, and vanilla. Bring to a simmer and cook for 5 to 6 minutes until the strawberries are soft. Use an immersion blender to purée the strawberries in the saucepan, or transfer the mixture to a blender and purée until smooth.

To make the waffles

1. In a medium bowl, whisk the flour, flaxseed, baking powder, baking soda, and salt until combined. Set the dry ingredients aside.

2. In a large bowl, whisk the canola oil, brown sugar, and cinnamon until well combined.

3. One at a time, whisk in the eggs until the mixture is fluffy.

4. Add the vanilla and milk, and whisk until combined.

5. Slowly whisk the dry ingredients into the wet ingredients.

6. Heat a Belgian waffle maker over medium heat. Once hot, coat with the cooking spray. Evenly spoon ⅔ cup of the batter into the waffle maker. Close the lid and cook for 1½ to 2 minutes until the waffle is browned on the outside. Repeat with the remaining batter.

7. Serve the waffles with the strawberry purée.

8. Once cooled, you can refrigerate the waffles in an airtight container or sealed plastic bag for up to five days. Serve chilled, or reheat in the microwave on high power for 30 seconds. Refrigerate the strawberry purée in a separate airtight container for up to five days.

COOKING TIP: To make the waffle batter into pancake batter, reduce the canola oil to 2 tablespoons and cook the same size portions in a greased nonstick skillet over medium heat for 1 to 2 minutes per side until set.

VARIATION TIP: Use raspberries or blueberries instead of strawberries to make the fruit purée.

PER SERVING: Calories: 381; Total Fat: 15g; Cholesterol: 106mg; Sodium: 459mg; Carbohydrates: 55g; Fiber: 9g; Protein: 12g

SPICY BAKED EGGS WITH GOAT CHEESE AND SPINACH

5-Ingredient, 30-Minute, Lower Calorie

Prep time: 5 minutes **Cook time:** 20 minutes **Total time:** 25 minutes

Baking eggs in a muffin tin or in ramekins is an easy way to feed several people at once. This recipe combines iron-rich spinach, spicy salsa for a little kick, and naturally low-fat goat cheese for richness and tang. ***Serves 4***

Nonstick cooking spray, for preparing the ramekins

10 ounces frozen chopped spinach, thawed and squeezed dry

4 large eggs

¼ cup chunky salsa

¼ cup crumbled goat cheese

Freshly ground black pepper

1. Preheat the oven to 325°F. Spray four (6-ounce) ramekins with cooking spray.

2. Cover the bottom of each ramekin with spinach. Make a slight indentation in the center of the spinach in each ramekin and crack an egg into it.

3. Top each egg with 1 tablespoon of salsa and 1 tablespoon of goat cheese. Season with pepper.

4. Place the ramekins on a baking sheet and bake for about 20 minutes, or until the whites are completely set but the yolks are still a bit runny. Serve immediately.

PER SERVING: Calories: 117; Total fat: 7g; Cholesterol: 191mg; Sodium: 250mg; Carbohydrates: 4g; Fiber: 3g; Protein: 9g

OVERNIGHT APPLE AND CHIA SEED REFRIGERATOR OATMEAL

Fertility Booster, Inflammation Fighter

Prep time: 5 minutes   **Total time:** 5 minutes, plus overnight chilling

Thanks to its high fiber content, oatmeal is an excellent whole-grain option for breakfast. Pair it with low-fat milk, Greek yogurt, apples, and chia seeds and you have a high-protein, satisfying breakfast loaded with antioxidants and calcium. As an added bonus, this oatmeal can stay in the refrigerator for up to 48 hours. ***Serves 1***

½ cup low-fat milk

½ cup low-fat plain Greek yogurt

¼ cup unsweetened applesauce

¼ cup old-fashioned rolled oats

1½ teaspoons chia seeds

⅛ teaspoon ground cinnamon

1. In a half-pint Mason jar, or any small container fitted with a lid, combine the milk, yogurt, applesauce, oats, chia seeds, and cinnamon.

2. Cover the jar and shake until well until combined. Refrigerate overnight and eat chilled the next day.

PREPARATION TIP: If you don't have either a Mason jar or a small container fitted with a lid, you can place all the ingredients in a small bowl, mix well, cover with plastic wrap, and chill overnight.

PER SERVING: Calories: 216; Total fat: 1g; Cholesterol: 7mg; Sodium: 10 mg; Carbohydrates: 37g; Fiber: 4g; Protein: 16g

MUSHROOM AND ASPARAGUS QUINOA FRITTATA

Fertility Booster, Inflammation Fighter

Prep time: 10 minutes **Cook time:** 30 minutes **Total time:** 40 minutes

Quinoa is an excellent source of fiber and protein. This recipe calls for cooked quinoa. You can find cooked quinoa in the frozen foods section of your grocery store. If you don't have cooked quinoa, use dried quinoa and prepare it according to the package directions. ***Serves 6***

2 teaspoons extra-virgin olive oil

1½ cups sliced mushrooms

1½ cups (1-inch) asparagus pieces

¼ teaspoon kosher salt, divided

1 cup chopped tomato

8 large eggs

4 large egg whites

½ cup low-fat milk

⅛ teaspoon freshly ground black pepper

1 cup cooked quinoa

½ cup shredded part-skim mozzarella cheese

1. Preheat the oven to 350°F and set the oven rack to the middle position.

2. In a medium oven-safe skillet or sauté pan, heat the olive oil over medium heat for 1 minute.

3. Add the mushrooms, asparagus, and ⅛ teaspoon of salt. Sauté for 5 to 6 minutes until the mushrooms are lightly browned and have released their moisture.

4. Add the tomato and cook 3 minutes more. Remove from the heat.

5. In a medium bowl, whisk the eggs, egg whites, milk, the remaining ⅛ teaspoon of salt, and the pepper.

6. Add the quinoa and cheese and stir until well combined. Add the egg mixture to the vegetables, gently stirring with a wooden spoon so the vegetables are evenly distributed.

7. Place the skillet on the middle rack and cook for 20 minutes, or until the egg mixture has set.

COOKING TIP: Want to change the taste profile of this dish? Add ¼ teaspoon of any of your favorite dried herbs while sautéing the vegetables to punch up the flavor. Suggestions include Salt-Free Italian Seasoning (page 139), herbes de Provence, curry powder, chili powder, cumin, and turmeric.

EQUIPMENT TIP: If you don't have an oven-safe skillet, transfer the vegetables and egg mixture to an 8-by-8-inch baking dish lightly coated with nonstick cooking spray.

PER SERVING: Calories: 207; Total fat: 10g; Cholesterol: 253mg; Sodium: 301mg; Carbohydrates: 11g; Fiber: 4g; Protein: 17g

RICOTTA TOAST WITH TOMATO AND CUCUMBER

30-Minute, Fertility Booster

Prep time: 5 minutes   **Total time:** 5 minutes

Sometimes a sweet breakfast just won't do. This toast hits the spot when you are in the mood for something a little savory. Ricotta is high in protein and contrasts nicely with the crunch of the toast and coolness of the cucumber. *Serves 1*

½ cup part-skim ricotta

1 tablespoon finely chopped scallion

¼ teaspoon Salt-Free Italian Seasoning (page 139)

⅛ teaspoon freshly ground black pepper

1 slice whole-grain or whole-wheat bread, toasted

1 small tomato, thinly sliced

¼ English cucumber, thinly sliced

1. In a small mixing bowl, combine the ricotta, scallion, Italian seasoning, and pepper. Using a rubber spatula, gently mix the ingredients to combine.

2. To assemble, spread the toast with the ricotta mixture and top with the tomato and cucumber slices. Serve immediately.

INGREDIENT TIP: Scallions are also known as green onions. If you don't have either, substitute an equal quantity of yellow or red onion.

PER SERVING: Calories: 274; Total fat: 11g; Cholesterol: 38mg; Sodium: 266mg; Carbohydrates: 27g; Fiber: 2g; Protein: 18g

SUPERFOOD GREEN SMOOTHIE

5-Ingredient, 30-Minute, Fertility Booster, Inflammation Fighter, Lower Calorie

Prep time: 5 minutes   **Total time:** 5 minutes

Creamy? Check. High in fiber? Absolutely. Delicious? You betcha!

Apple, avocado, kale, and spinach give this cold drink the taste of tangy fresh greens with just the right amount of sweetness. This recipe, which I adapted from *The DASH Diet for Beginners: The Guide to Getting Started*, is still chock-full of fiber and heart-healthy fats. This tasty smoothie is sure to energize your morning. ***Serves 1***

1 cup coarsely chopped kale leaves

1 cup fresh spinach leaves

1 medium Hass avocado, pitted and coarsely chopped

½ medium apple, peeled and coarsely chopped

½ to ¾ cup cold water

2 tablespoons freshly squeezed lemon

2 or 3 ice cubes

1. In a blender, combine the kale, spinach, avocado, and apple and process until smooth.

2. Slowly add the water, lemon juice, and ice and pulse until puréed. Serve immediately.

PREPARATION TIP: Change the amount of water and ice to suit how thick or thin you prefer your smoothies. For a thinner smoothie, add more water and less ice. For a thicker smoothie, you can decrease the amount of water and increase the amount of ice.

PER SERVING: Calories: 167; Total fat: 6g; Cholesterol: 0mg; Sodium: 99mg; Carbohydrates: 14g; Fiber: 7g; Protein: 11g

PINEAPPLE-BANANA HIGH-PROTEIN SMOOTHIE

5-Ingredient, 30-Minute, Fertility Booster, Inflammation Fighter

Prep time: 5 minutes **Total time:** 5 minutes

Pineapples are low in calories and a great source of vitamins, minerals, and antioxidants. They are rich in vitamins A and C and are particularly high in an enzyme called bromelain. Bromelain is a powerful inflammation fighter and aids in digestion. Cheers to your health! *Serves 1*

½ cup fresh or frozen pineapple cubes
½ medium banana
½ cup low-fat plain Greek yogurt
¼ medium Hass avocado, peeled, pitted, and
  coarsely chopped

½ to ¾ cup low-fat milk
2 or 3 ice cubes

1. In a blender, combine the pineapple, banana, yogurt, and avocado. Process until smooth.
2. Slowly add the milk and ice and pulse until puréed. Serve immediately.

PREPARATION TIP: Add more water and less ice if you prefer a thinner smoothie. Or go for a thicker smoothie, with less water and more ice.

PER SERVING: Calories: 246; Total fat: 5g; Cholesterol: 7mg; Sodium: 106mg; Carbohydrates: 37g; Fiber: 6g; Protein: 15g

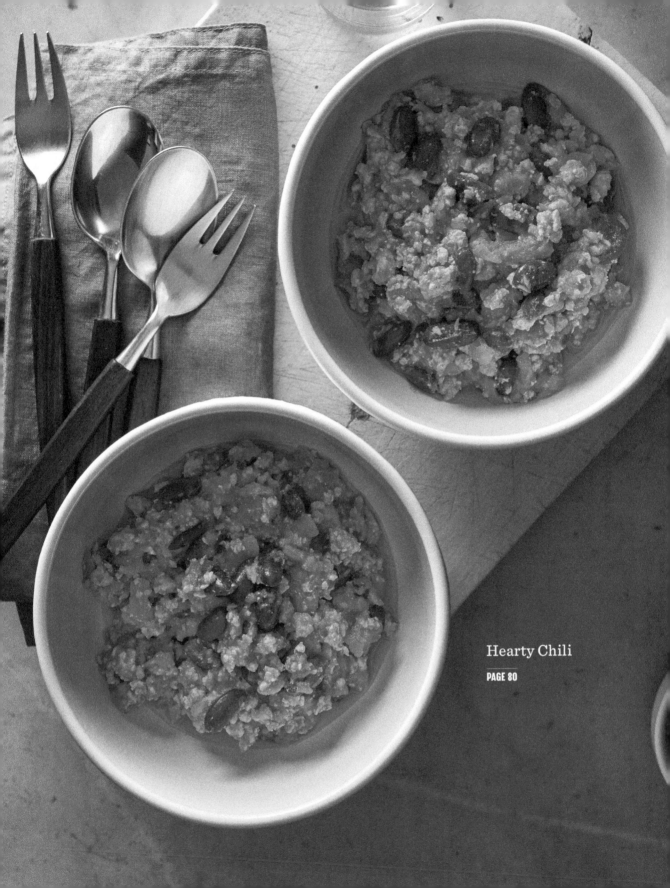

Hearty Chili

PAGE 80

5.
SALADS, SOUPS, AND MORE

THREE-BEAN VEGETABLE SALAD

Fertility Booster, Inflammation Fighter

Prep time: 15 minutes   **Total time:** 15 minutes, plus 1 hour to chill

Hearty, high in fiber, and sure to be a fiesta in your mouth, this colorful three-bean vegetable salad makes a perfect lunch or light dinner served on a bed of shredded lettuce. ***Serves 6***

FOR THE SALAD DRESSING

½ cup red wine vinegar

¼ cup extra-virgin olive oil

2 tablespoons freshly squeezed lime juice

1 tablespoon freshly squeezed lemon juice

1 garlic clove, minced

¼ cup chopped fresh cilantro

2 teaspoons ground cumin

2 teaspoons freshly ground black pepper

¼ teaspoon chili powder

Dash hot sauce

FOR THE BEAN SALAD

1 (16-ounce) can low-sodium black beans, rinsed well and drained

1 (16-ounce) can low-sodium kidney beans, rinsed well and drained

1 (16-ounce) can low-sodium cannellini beans, rinsed well and drained

1 medium green bell pepper, chopped

1 medium red bell pepper, chopped

1 (10-ounce) package frozen organic corn, thawed

1 cup chopped red onion

To make the salad dressing

> In a small bowl, combine the vinegar, olive oil, lime and lemon juices, garlic, cilantro, cumin, pepper, chili powder, and hot sauce. Whisk until smooth. Set aside.

To make the bean salad

1. In a large bowl, stir together the black, kidney, and cannellini beans, green and red bell peppers, corn, and red onion.

2. Pour the dressing over the vegetables. Using a rubber spatula, mix until the ingredients are well distributed. Chill for at least 1 hour before serving over a bed of lettuce.

MAKE-AHEAD TIP: Refrigerate in an airtight container for up to five days.

PER SERVING: Calories: 260; Total fat: 4g; Cholesterol: 0mg; Sodium: 345mg; Carbohydrates: 48g; Fiber: 11g; Protein: 13g

FENNEL-APPLE-WALNUT SALAD

30-Minute, Fertility Booster, Inflammation Fighter, Lower Calorie

Prep time: 10 minutes   **Total time:** 10 minutes

Fennel is high in vitamin C and fiber. It has a mild, sweet flavor and is a great addition to any dish. When buying fennel look for a firm white bulb, bright green leaves, and an unblemished stalk. Although this recipe only uses the bulb, all parts of the fennel plant are edible. *Serves 6*

8 cups salad greens of choice

1 medium fennel bulb, trimmed and thinly sliced

2 medium apples, peeled, cored, quartered, and thinly sliced

6 tablespoons goat cheese, divided

6 tablespoons walnuts, divided

6 tablespoons apple cider vinegar, divided

12 teaspoons extra-virgin olive oil, divided

Freshly ground black pepper

1. Divide the salad greens among six small salad plates.
2. Equally divide the fennel and apple slices and distribute them over the greens.
3. Sprinkle each salad with 1 tablespoon of goat cheese and 1 tablespoon of walnuts.
4. Drizzle each salad with 1 tablespoon of vinegar and 2 teaspoons of olive oil. Season with pepper and serve immediately.

PREPARATION TIP: If you want to prepare this salad ahead, prepare through step 3. Dress the salad with the vinegar and olive oil just before serving so the greens don't get soggy.

PER SERVING: Calories: 176; Total fat: 10g; Cholesterol: 13mg; Sodium: 112mg; Carbohydrates: 10g; Fiber: 2g; Protein: 6g

QUINOA AND BLACK BEAN BOWLS WITH CILANTRO VINAIGRETTE

Fertility Booster, Inflammation Fighter

Prep time: 15 minutes **Cook time:** 20 minutes **Total time:** 35 minutes

Who doesn't love a good bowl? This recipe certainly delivers on the goodness, with hot quinoa topped with black beans and roasted vegetables, and then drizzled with personality-filled cilantro vinaigrette. Talk about an all-star nutrient lineup! *Serves 6*

FOR THE BEAN BOWLS

1½ cups thinly sliced red bell pepper

1½ cups thinly sliced green bell pepper

1 small onion, thinly sliced

1 tablespoon extra-virgin olive oil

1 teaspoon chili powder

½ teaspoon garlic powder

½ teaspoon ground cumin

½ teaspoon smoked paprika

½ teaspoon onion powder

⅛ teaspoon kosher salt

2 tablespoons freshly squeezed lime juice

1½ cups cooked quinoa

1 (16-ounce) can low-sodium black beans, rinsed well and drained

1½ cups shredded iceberg lettuce

1½ cups chopped tomatoes

FOR THE CILANTRO VINAIGRETTE

2 cups packed fresh cilantro with stems

1 avocado, pitted and coarsely chopped

3 to 4 garlic cloves, minced

¼ cup extra-virgin olive oil

¼ cup water

2 tablespoons red wine vinegar

Kosher salt

Freshly ground black pepper

To make the bean bowls

1. Preheat the oven to 425°F. Line a rimmed baking sheet with parchment paper or aluminum foil. Set aside.

2. In a large bowl, combine the red and green bell peppers, onion, olive oil, chili powder, garlic powder, cumin, paprika, onion powder, and salt. Using a rubber spatula, mix until well combined and the vegetables are coated in the oil and seasonings. Pour vegetable mixture onto the prepared baking sheet. Roast for 20 minutes.

3. In a medium bowl, stir together the lime juice and cooked quinoa. Set aside.

To make the cilantro vinaigrette

In a blender or food processor, combine the cilantro, avocado, garlic, olive oil, water, and vinegar. Blend until smooth. Season with salt and pepper.

To assemble the bowls

In each of six bowls, place ¼ cup cooked quinoa. Top the quinoa with ⅓ cup black beans, about ½ cup vegetable mixture, ¼ cup lettuce, and ¼ cup tomatoes. Drizzle each bowl with 2 tablespoons of cilantro vinaigrette.

PREPARATION TIP: Buy boil-in-bag brown quinoa or precooked quinoa sold in the freezer section of your grocery store to save time without skimping on nutrients.

PER SERVING: Calories: 350; Total fat: 13g; Cholesterol: 0mg; Sodium: 281mg; Carbohydrates: 39g; Fiber: 10g; Protein: 12g

FRENCH LENTIL SALAD

Fertility Booster, Inflammation Fighter, Lower Calorie

Prep time: 10 minutes   **Cook time:** 40 minutes, plus 1 hour to chill   **Total time:** 1 hour, 50 minutes

This is a perfect make-ahead lunch. It's inexpensive, high in fiber, filling, and simple to make. In fact, the flavors intensify the longer you allow the lentils to soak up the vinaigrette. If you are looking for a little more bulk, add some diced cucumbers or bell peppers to the salad. ***Serves 6***

FOR THE LENTILS

1 tablespoon extra-virgin olive oil

1 cup finely chopped onion

1 medium celery stalk, finely chopped

1 medium carrot, finely chopped

3 garlic cloves, minced

1 teaspoon mustard seed

1 teaspoon fennel seed

½ cup water

2 cups Homemade Vegetable Broth (page 140), or store-bought low-sodium vegetable broth, or low-sodium chicken broth

1 cup green lentils, picked through, rinsed well, and drained

1 tablespoon chopped fresh thyme leaves, or 1 teaspoon dried thyme

2 dried bay leaves

FOR THE VINAIGRETTE

1 tablespoon red wine vinegar

1 tablespoon Dijon mustard

¼ cup cooking liquid from lentils

FOR THE LENTIL SALAD

1 cup cherry tomatoes, halved

2 tablespoons fresh parsley, cut into strips, or 1 teaspoon dried parsley

Kosher salt

Freshly ground black pepper

8 cups lettuce of choice

To make the lentils

1. In a large saucepan, heat the olive oil over medium heat. Add the onion, celery, and carrot. Sauté for 5 to 6 minutes until the vegetables are soft.

2. Add the garlic, mustard seed, and fennel seed. Sauté for about 1 minute, or until the herbs become fragrant.

3. Add the water, vegetable broth, lentils, thyme, and bay leaves. Increase the heat to high and bring the mixture to a boil. Boil for 1 minute. Cover the pan, decrease the heat to low, and simmer for about 25 to 30 minutes, or until the lentils are firm but fairly tender.

4. Drain the lentils, reserving ¼ cup of cooking liquid. Pour the lentils into a large bowl. Remove and discard the bay leaves. Refrigerate the lentils for about 1 hour to chill.

To make the vinaigrette

In a small bowl, whisk the vinegar, mustard, and reserved cooking liquid. Set aside.

To assemble the lentil salad

Once the lentils have cooled, add the vinaigrette, tomatoes, and parsley. Gently toss to coat. Season with salt and pepper. Serve chilled over a bed of lettuce.

PER SERVING: (½ cup cooked lentils) Calories: 189; Total fat: 5g; Cholesterol: 2mg; Sodium: 185mg; Carbohydrates: 25g; Fiber: 11g; Protein: 11g

HEARTY CHILI

Fertility Booster, Inflammation Fighter

Prep time: 15 minutes   **Cook time:** 1 hour, 15 minutes   **Total time:** 1 hour, 30 minutes

Both meat and nonmeat eaters alike love chili. This recipe can be easily adapted into a meatless version by simply omitting the ground beef. No matter what your eating style, each version is loaded with veggies, high in fiber, and contains plenty of protein to satisfy just about anyone's taste buds. ***Serves 6***

1 tablespoon extra-virgin olive oil

1 medium onion, diced

2 garlic cloves, minced

1 cup chopped green bell pepper

1 cup chopped red bell pepper

1 pound 93% lean ground beef (optional)

1 (28-ounce) can no-salt-added diced tomatoes

1 (16-ounce) can low-sodium black beans, rinsed well and drained

1 (16-ounce) can low-sodium kidney beans, rinsed well and drained

2 tablespoons chili powder

2 tablespoons paprika

1 teaspoon freshly ground black pepper

2½ cups frozen mixed vegetables (a blend of carrots, broccoli, cauliflower)

¾ cup shredded low-fat Cheddar cheese, divided

Low-fat plain Greek yogurt, for garnish (optional)

1. In a Dutch oven or a large soup pot, heat the olive oil over medium-high heat. Add the onion and garlic and cook for 1 to 2 minutes until the onion is translucent. Decrease the heat to medium.

2. Add the green and red bell peppers and cook for 3 to 4 minutes more until softened.

3. Add the ground beef (if using). Cook for 7 to 10 minutes, stirring the meat occasionally while it cooks and breaking up large chunks with the back of a spoon.

4. Stir in the tomatoes, black beans, kidney beans, chili powder, paprika, and black pepper. Decrease the heat and simmer for 5 to 7 minutes.

5. While the chili simmers, put the mixed vegetables in a food processor or blender and pulse 4 to 5 times into bite-size pieces. Transfer the vegetables to the chili. Continue to simmer for 30 to 45 minutes.

6. Serve warm. Garnish each serving with 2 tablespoons of shredded cheese and a dollop of yogurt (if using).

PER SERVING: (with 2 tablespoons cheese and lean ground beef) Calories: 330; Total fat: 9g; Cholesterol: 49mg; Sodium: 380mg; Carbohydrates: 35g; Fiber: 9g; Protein: 28g

PER SERVING: (with 2 tablespoons cheese, but no ground beef) Calories: 220; Total fat: 3g; Cholesterol: 18mg; Sodium: 320mg; Carbohydrates: 35g; Fiber: 9g; Protein: 14g

VEGETABLE AND WHITE BEAN SOUP

Fertility Booster, Inflammation Fighter

Prep time: 15 minutes **Cook time:** 35 minutes **Total time:** 50 minutes

There is nothing quite like a hot bowl of healthy soup to ward off a chill. This recipe includes a rainbow of vegetables and is chock-full of vitamins, minerals, antioxidants, fiber, and protein. A hearty dollop of pesto makes an excellent finish for this soup. ***Serves 6***

2 tablespoons extra-virgin olive oil

1 large onion, chopped

3 garlic cloves, minced

3 medium carrots, chopped

2 celery stalks, chopped

8 cups Homemade Vegetable Broth (page 140), or store-bought low-sodium vegetable broth, or low-sodium chicken broth

3 cups (½-inch pieces) fresh green beans

2 (16-ounce) cans low-sodium cannellini beans, or other white beans, rinsed well and drained

4 Roma tomatoes, seeded and roughly chopped

2 medium zucchini, chopped

4 cups chopped kale or collard greens, hard ribs removed

2 teaspoons red wine vinegar

¼ teaspoon kosher salt

½ teaspoon freshly ground black pepper

6 teaspoons Basil Pesto (page 136; optional)

1. In a large soup pot, heat the olive oil over medium-high heat. Add the onion and garlic, cooking for 1 to 2 minutes until the onion is translucent. Add the carrots and celery. Cook for 8 to 10 minutes, stirring frequently, until the vegetables begin to soften.

2. Add the broth and bring to a boil.

3. Add the green beans. Decrease the heat to a low simmer and cook, stirring occasionally, until the vegetables are soft, 13 to 15 minutes.

4. Stir in the cannellini beans, tomatoes, zucchini, kale, vinegar, salt, and pepper. Increase the heat to medium; cook the soup for 10 to 12 minutes until the zucchini and kale have softened.

5. Ladle into warmed bowls and top each serving with 1 teaspoon of pesto (if using).

INGREDIENT TIP: If you don't have kale or collard greens, substitute fresh spinach.

PER SERVING: (2 cups) Calories: 225; Total fat: 8g; Cholesterol: 0mg; Sodium: 325mg; Carbohydrates: 28g; Fiber: 8g; Protein: 13g

VEGETABLE AND HUMMUS PITA

30-Minute, Lower Calorie

Prep time: 5 minutes **Total time:** 5 minutes

Vegetarians worldwide are intimate with salad stuffed in a pita and slathered with lemony hummus. Endlessly versatile, this is an excellent way to pile on the vegetables, get a nice hit of protein, and deliver it all in a convenient pita, which is a much healthier choice than most commercially made breads. ***Serves 4***

1 cup Homemade Hummus (page 137)

¼ cup chopped fresh basil, or parsley

1 tablespoon lemon zest

1 tablespoon extra-virgin olive oil

Freshly ground black pepper

2 whole-wheat pitas, split

2 cups chopped red leaf lettuce, romaine lettuce, or butter lettuce

2 medium carrots, shredded

1 cucumber, thinly sliced

1 red onion, thinly sliced

1 large tomato, thinly sliced

1. In a small bowl, stir together the hummus, basil, lemon zest, and olive oil. Season with pepper and mix until smooth.

2. Spread a few tablespoons of hummus on the inside of each pita. Tuck some of the lettuce, carrots, cucumber, red onion, and tomato into each pita. Drizzle additional hummus into the center of the vegetables, if desired, and serve.

INGREDIENT TIP: You can substitute plain store-bought hummus for the homemade version to save some time.

PER SERVING: Calories: 168; Total fat: 11g; Cholesterol: 0g; Sodium: 437mg; Carbohydrates: 38g; Fiber: 9g; Protein: 10g

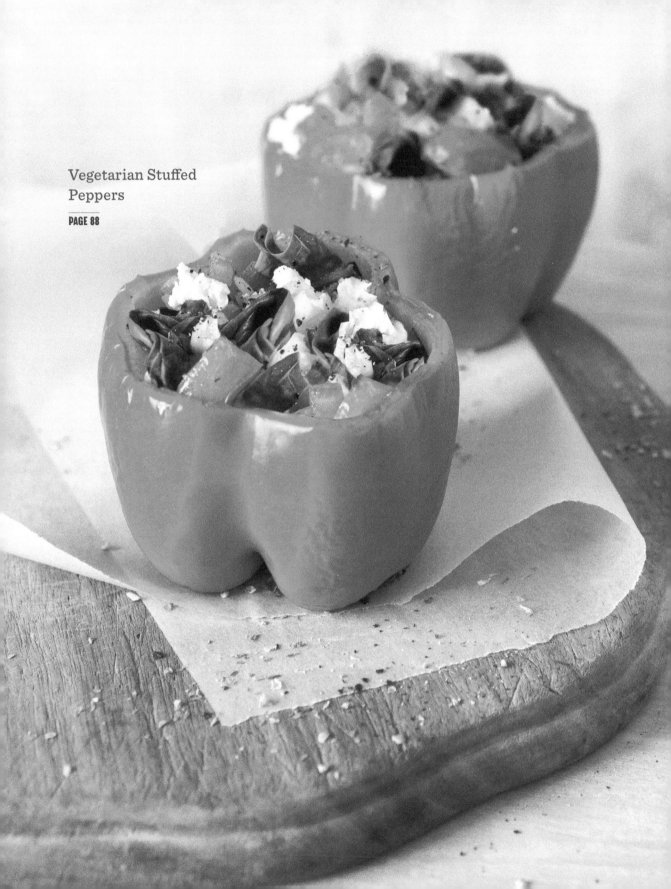

Vegetarian Stuffed
Peppers

PAGE 88

6.
MEATLESS MAINS

SWEET POTATO AND BLACK BEAN TORTILLAS WITH AVOCADO YOGURT SAUCE

Fertility Booster, Inflammation Fighter

Prep time: 15 minutes   **Cook time:** 20 minutes   **Total time:** 35 minutes

Whole-wheat tortillas are the perfect vehicle for delivering a dose of heart-healthy fat, fiber, protein, and calcium. These sweet potato–filled tortillas are hearty, creamy, tangy, and bursting with fresh flavors. They are an easy, inexpensive, and delicious option when you need a quick dinner the whole family will enjoy. ***Serves 6***

FOR THE FILLING

2 medium sweet potatoes, peeled and cubed

1 tablespoon extra-virgin olive oil

½ teaspoon chili powder

½ teaspoon ground cumin

⅛ teaspoon kosher salt

⅛ teaspoon freshly ground black pepper

6 medium whole-wheat tortillas

3 cups shredded romaine lettuce

1 cup seeded and diced tomato

4 scallions, thinly sliced

1½ cups low-sodium canned beans of choice, rinsed well and drained

Fresh lime wedges, for serving (optional)

FOR THE AVOCADO YOGURT SAUCE

½ cup low-fat plain Greek yogurt

1 medium Hass avocado, peeled and pitted

2 tablespoons freshly squeezed lime juice

1 garlic clove, minced

Kosher salt

Freshly ground black pepper

To make the filling

1. Preheat the oven to 400°F. Line a large baking sheet with parchment paper or aluminum foil. Set aside.

2. In a large bowl, toss together the sweet potatoes, olive oil, chili powder, cumin, salt, and pepper. Spread the sweet potatoes in a single layer on the prepared baking sheet. Bake for 20 minutes, or until fork-tender.

To make the avocado yogurt sauce

While the sweet potatoes roast, in a food processor or blender, combine the yogurt, avocado, lime juice, garlic, and a pinch salt and pepper. Process until smooth. Refrigerate until needed.

To assemble the tortillas

On top of the tortillas, evenly distribute the lettuce, tomatoes, and scallions. To each tortilla add ⅙ of the roasted sweet potatoes and ¼ cup black beans. Drizzle with the avocado yogurt sauce and a squeeze of fresh lime juice (if using). Fold in half to eat.

PER SERVING: (1 tortilla) Calories: 315; Total fat: 8g; Cholesterol: 2mg; Sodium: 330mg; Carbohydrates: 45g; Fiber: 12g; Protein: 13g

VEGETARIAN STUFFED PEPPERS

Fertility Booster, Inflammation Fighter

Prep time: 15 minutes **Cook time:** 30 minutes **Total time:** 45 minutes

These easy vegetarian stuffed peppers are loaded with veggies, fiber, protein, and a blend of Mexican spices. If you like some heat in your food, before cooking the peppers, add a dash of your favorite hot sauce to the rice mixture. ***Serves 6***

Nonstick cooking spray, for preparing the baking dish

1 tablespoon extra-virgin olive oil

1 cup chopped onion

¼ cup spinach, raw

2 garlic cloves, minced

6 whole large red bell peppers, seeded, membranes removed, tops removed and chopped

3 cups cooked brown rice

1 (16-ounce) can low-sodium black beans, rinsed well and drained

1 (14.5-ounce) can no-salt-added petite-diced tomatoes, drained

1½ teaspoons chili powder

1½ teaspoons ground cumin

¾ cup low-fat shredded Cheddar cheese

1. Preheat the oven to 350°F. Coat a 9-by-13-inch baking dish with cooking spray. Set aside.

2. In a large skillet, heat the olive oil over medium heat.

3. Add the onion, spinach, and garlic and cook for 1 to 2 minutes until the onion is translucent.

4. Add the chopped pepper tops and sauté for 5 to 7 minutes until tender. Transfer the cooked vegetables to a large bowl.

5. Add the cooked rice, black beans, tomatoes, chili powder, and cumin. Using a rubber spatula, mix the ingredients well.

6. Add the cheese and mix until it's evenly distributed throughout the rice mixture. Spoon the rice mixture into each bell pepper and arrange the filled peppers in the prepared baking dish.

7. Bake for 30 minutes. Serve warm.

PER SERVING: (1 stuffed pepper) Calories: 402; Total fat: 4g; Cholesterol: 8mg; Sodium: 285mg; Carbohydrates: 43g; Fiber: 8g; Protein: 13g

CREAMY LENTILS WITH KALE, SPINACH, AND ARTICHOKE HEARTS

30-Minute, Fertility Booster, Inflammation Fighter

Prep time: 10 minutes **Cook time:** 20 minutes **Total time:** 30 minutes

Many people consider kale one of the healthiest foods on the planet. It is low in calories, high in vitamins and minerals, and contains many disease-fighting antioxidants. The lentils and artichoke make it an especially satisfying meatless dish. Red lentils cook the quickest; you'll need to cook green or brown lentils longer for them to achieve the same tenderness. I toss spinach into the mix and round out the flavors with Parmesan cheese. *Serves 6*

1¾ cups Homemade Vegetable Broth (page 140), or store-bought low-sodium vegetable broth

¾ cup dried red lentils, picked through, rinsed well, and drained

¼ teaspoon dried oregano

⅛ teaspoon freshly ground black pepper

1¾ tablespoons extra-virgin olive oil

4 garlic cloves, minced

8 cups loosely packed chopped kale

4 cups fresh spinach leaves

2 (9-ounce) boxes frozen artichoke hearts, thawed

¾ teaspoon Salt-Free Italian Seasoning (page 139)

2 tablespoons grated Parmesan cheese

1½ cups cooked brown rice, warm

1. In a medium saucepan over high heat, combine the vegetable broth, lentils, oregano, and pepper and bring to a boil. Reduce the heat to low, cover the saucepan, and simmer for 12 to 15 minutes, or until the lentils have absorbed most of the broth and are tender. Remove from the heat.

2. In a medium skillet, warm the olive oil and garlic over medium heat.

3. Add the kale and spinach and cook for 4 to 5 minutes until wilted.

4. Stir in the artichoke hearts and Italian seasoning. Cook for 3 to 5 minutes, or until the artichokes are warmed through. Remove from the heat and stir in the Parmesan cheese.

5. To serve, layer the lentils and kale mixture over the brown rice.

PER SERVING: Calories: 241; Total fat: 3g; Cholesterol: 2mg; Sodium: 178mg; Carbohydrates: 42g; Fiber: 14g; Protein: 14g

PASTA PRIMAVERA

30-Minute, Fertility Booster, Inflammation Fighter

Prep time: 10 minutes   **Cook time:** 20 minutes   **Total time:** 30 minutes

Traditionally a dish made in the spring and summer months, this easy, veggie-packed meal is delicious year-round. Unlike the traditional version, this recipe has no cream, but instead, uses fat-free evaporated milk to add body to the sauce without the extra calories, fat, and sodium. Experiment with different seasonal vegetables, aiming for about 5 to 6 cups of fresh raw veggies to start, and various types of whole-wheat pasta to find the combinations you like best. ***Serves 6***

1 cup fresh asparagus, trimmed and cut into
　2-inch pieces

1 cup (¼-inch rounds) sliced yellow squash

1 cup sliced red bell pepper

1 cup sliced green bell pepper

1 cup cherry tomatoes, halved

1 tablespoon extra-virgin olive oil

2 garlic cloves, minced

½ cup chopped onion

1 teaspoon unsalted butter

1 cup low-fat evaporated milk

Zest of 1 lemon

½ cup grated Parmesan cheese

12 ounces whole-wheat pasta

2 teaspoons Salt-Free Italian Seasoning (page 139)

1. Place a steamer basket into a large pot and fill the pot with about 1 inch of water. Bring the water to a boil over high heat. To the steamer basket, add the asparagus, squash, red and green bell peppers, and tomatoes. Cover and steam for 8 minutes, or until the tomatoes start to soften. Remove the vegetables from the pot and set aside.

2. In a large saucepan, heat the olive oil over medium heat. Add the garlic and onion and sauté for 1 to 2 minutes until the onion is translucent. Add the steamed vegetables and toss to combine. Remove from the heat but keep warm.

3. In another large saucepan over medium heat, combine the butter, evaporated milk, lemon zest, and Parmesan cheese. Cook, stirring continuously to avoid scalding, until thickened. Remove from the heat and cover the pan with a lid.

4. Meanwhile, fill a large 6-quart pot about three-fourths full of water and bring it to a boil over high heat. Add the pasta and cook for about 9 to 12 minutes, or according to the package directions. Drain the pasta.

5. Distribute the pasta evenly among six plates. Top each serving of pasta with the vegetable mixture. Evenly spoon the sauce over each dish. Season with the Salt-Free Italian Seasoning and serve immediately.

PER SERVING: Calories: 320; Total fat: 6g; Cholesterol: 8mg; Sodium: 168mg; Carbohydrates: 54g; Fiber: 3g; Protein: 15g

ROASTED TOMATO AND BARLEY RISOTTO

Fertility Booster, Inflammation Fighter

Prep time: 10 minutes   **Cook time:** 1 hour, 15 minutes   **Total time:** 1 hour, 25 minutes

There are two types of barley—hulled and pearl. This recipe uses pearl barley to save time. It is slightly more processed than hulled barley, and it doesn't require an overnight presoak. Don't worry, though; pearl barley remains a good source of fiber, potassium, calcium, and magnesium, making it a heart-healthy whole grain. **Serves 6**

Nonstick cooking spray, for preparing the baking sheet

3 cups cherry tomatoes, halved

2 tablespoons extra-virgin olive oil, divided

Kosher salt

Freshly ground black pepper

3 cups Homemade Vegetable Broth (page 140), or store-bought low-sodium vegetable broth

2¼ cups water

1 medium onion, finely chopped

2 cloves minced garlic

1½ cups dry pearl barley

1½ tablespoons chopped fresh thyme leaves

3 tablespoons chopped fresh parsley

3 tablespoons chopped fresh basil

½ cup grated Parmesan cheese

1. Preheat the oven to 350°F. Lightly coat a rimmed baking sheet with nonstick cooking spray. Set aside.

2. In a medium bowl, gently toss the tomatoes with 1 tablespoon of olive oil and a pinch salt and pepper.

3. Transfer the tomatoes to the baking sheet and roast for 12 to 13 minutes, or until their skin starts to wrinkle.

4. In a 6-quart saucepan over high heat, bring the vegetable broth and water to a boil. Decrease the heat to low and simmer.

5. In an 8-quart saucepan, heat the remaining 1 tablespoon of olive oil over medium heat. Add the onion and garlic and cook for 1 to 2 minutes until the onion is translucent.

6. Stir in the barley and cook for 2 minutes, stirring continuously.

7. In ½-cup increments, pour the broth mixture into the barley and cook until completely absorbed, stirring occasionally to ensure the barley doesn't stick to the bottom of the pan. Each time you add the broth mixture make sure the liquid is completely absorbed before adding more. Cook until the barley becomes tender, about 45 to 50 minutes total. Remove the barley from the heat. Carefully fold in the roasted tomatoes, thyme, parsley, fresh basil, and Parmesan cheese.

8. Equally portion the risotto among six shallow bowls and serve immediately.

PER SERVING: Calories: 281; Total fat: 8g; Cholesterol: 7mg; Sodium: 160mg; Carbohydrates: 46g; Fiber: 10g; Protein: 10g

VEGETABLE MOO SHU WRAPS

30-Minute, Fertility Booster, Inflammation Fighter

Prep time: 5 minutes **Cook time:** 10 minutes **Total time:** 15 minutes

The use of bagged shredded vegetables means this dish can be on the table in no time. And the substitution of whole-wheat tortillas for traditional wraps boosts the fiber and nutritional content of this healthy meal. *Serves 4*

3 teaspoons sesame oil, divided

4 large eggs, lightly beaten

2 teaspoons peeled and minced fresh ginger

2 garlic cloves, minced

1 (12-ounce) bag shredded coleslaw mix, or broccoli slaw

2 cups bean sprouts

1 bunch scallions, sliced, divided

1 tablespoon low-sodium soy sauce

1 tablespoon unseasoned rice vinegar

2 tablespoons hoisin sauce

4 whole-wheat tortillas, warmed according to the package directions

1. In a large nonstick skillet, heat 1 teaspoon of sesame oil over medium heat. Add the eggs and cook, stirring, for about 3 minutes until just set. Transfer the eggs to a plate.

2. In the same skillet, heat the remaining 2 teaspoons of sesame oil over medium heat. Add the ginger and garlic and cook for 1 minute.

3. Stir in the coleslaw mix, bean sprouts, half the scallions, the soy sauce, and vinegar. Cover the skillet and cook for about 3 minutes until the vegetables are tender.

4. Return the cooked eggs to the skillet. Stir in the hoisin sauce and cook, stirring, for about 2 minutes. Remove from the heat and add the remaining scallions.

5. Place the warm tortillas on serving plates and divide the vegetable mixture among them. Tightly roll up each tortilla around the veggies and serve immediately.

PER SERVING: Calories: 216; Total fat: 10g; Cholesterol: 186mg; Sodium: 461mg; Carbohydrates: 23g; Fiber: 5g; Protein: 11g

VEGETARIAN SPAGHETTI SQUASH CASSEROLE

Fertility Booster, Inflammation Fighter

Prep time: 20 minutes   **Cook time:** 1 hour, 25 minutes   **Total time:** 1 hour, 45 minutes

This is a low-carbohydrate dish full of flavor that everyone is sure to enjoy. The ricotta and mozzarella cheese deliver protein, calcium, and vitamin D, and the squash, spinach, mushrooms, and tomatoes are a great source of fiber and antioxidants, making this a nutrient-packed dish. Pair it with a simple salad for the perfect weeknight meal. *Serves 6*

Nonstick cooking spray, for preparing the baking sheet
2 medium spaghetti squash (about 4 pounds total)
Kosher salt
Freshly ground black pepper
2 teaspoons extra-virgin olive oil
1 medium onion, chopped
2 cups chopped mushrooms
2 garlic cloves, minced
1½ cups part-skim ricotta

1½ cups chopped fresh spinach
1 large egg white (optional)
⅓ cup grated Parmesan cheese
2 teaspoons Salt-Free Italian Seasoning (page 139)
2 large Roma tomatoes, chopped
½ cup no-salt-added crushed tomatoes
¼ cup shredded part-skim mozzarella cheese
⅛ teaspoon red pepper flakes

1. Preheat the oven to 400°F. Coat a rimmed baking sheet with cooking spray. Set aside.

2. With a sharp knife, carefully halve the spaghetti squash vertically. Using a spoon, remove and discard the seeds and membranes. Season the flesh with salt and pepper. Place the squash halves, cut-side down, on the prepared baking sheet and bake for 1 hour, or until soft. Set aside and let cool.

3. Turn the oven temperature to 350°F.

4. While the squash bakes, in a medium sauté pan or skillet, heat the olive oil over medium heat.

5. Add the onion and cook for 1 to 2 minutes until it is translucent. Add the mushrooms and garlic and continue to cook until the mushrooms have released most of their moisture and are golden brown, 6 to 7 minutes more. Drain any remaining moisture and set aside.

6. In a large bowl, gently stir together the ricotta, spinach, egg white, Parmesan cheese, and Italian seasoning.

CONTINUED >>

7. Fold in the mushroom and onion mixture.

8. Add the Roma tomatoes and stir until well combined. Season with salt and pepper. Set aside until the squash is cool enough to handle.

9. Once the squash has cooled and you are able to handle it safely, use a fork to separate the flesh into spaghetti-like strands. Discard the squash skin.

10. Lightly coat a 9-by-13-inch baking dish with cooking spray. Fill the bottom of the dish with the spaghetti squash. Top with the ricotta and mushroom mixture. Add a thin layer of crushed tomatoes. Sprinkle with the mozzarella cheese and red pepper flakes. Bake for 20 to 25 minutes, or until the cheese is bubbly.

PER SERVING: Calories: 219; Total fat: 11g; Cholesterol: 18mg; Sodium: 248mg; Carbohydrates: 18g; Fiber: 3g; Protein: 13g

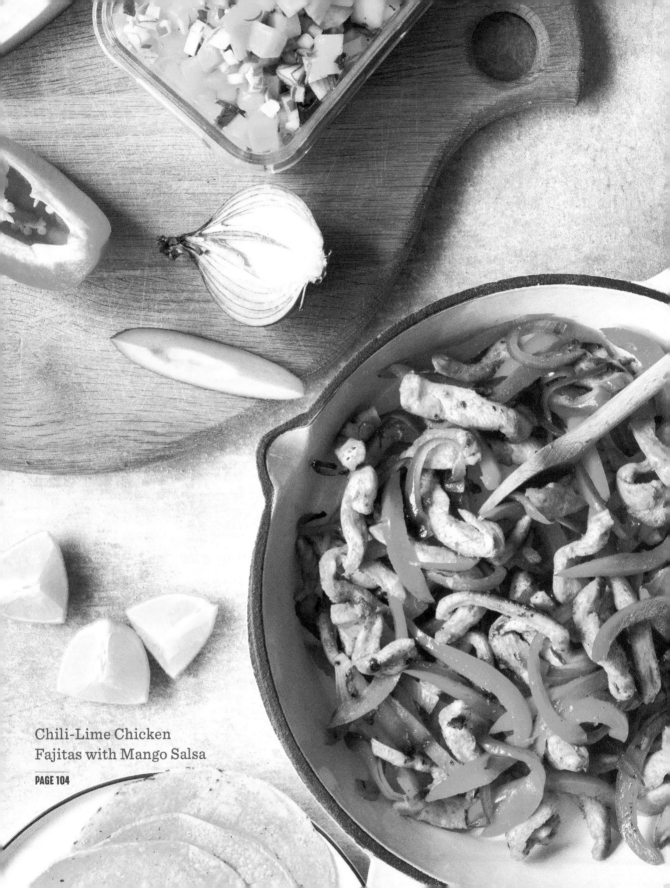

Chili-Lime Chicken
Fajitas with Mango Salsa

PAGE 104

7.
POULTRY AND SEAFOOD MAINS

TURKEY-STUFFED PEPPERS

Inflammation Fighter

Prep time: 15 minutes **Cook time:** 45 minutes **Total time:** 1 hour

These stuffed peppers are a perfect complete meal. They combine a lean protein, a serving of vegetables, and a whole-grain carbohydrate. If you are looking to bring down the calories and carbohydrates, substitute cooked cauliflower rice for the brown rice.
Serves 3

Nonstick cooking spray, for preparing the baking dish
2 teaspoons extra-virgin olive oil
1 cup chopped onion
1 garlic clove, minced
2 tablespoons chopped fresh parsley
1 pound 93% lean ground turkey
1 teaspoon garlic powder
1 teaspoon ground cumin

⅛ teaspoon kosher salt
Freshly ground black pepper
½ cup no-salt-added tomato sauce
1 cup low-sodium chicken broth, divided
3 large red bell peppers, halved, seeded, and
 membranes removed
1½ cups cooked brown rice
6 tablespoons shredded low-fat Cheddar cheese

1. Preheat the oven to 400°F. Lightly coat a 9-by-13-inch baking dish with cooking spray. Set aside.

2. In a medium skillet, heat the olive oil over medium heat.

3. Add the onion, garlic, and parsley. Cook for 1 to 2 minutes until the onion is translucent.

4. Add the ground turkey, garlic powder, cumin, and salt. Season with pepper. Cook for 6 to 8 minutes, breaking up any large chunks of meat with the back of a wooden spoon, or until the meat is completely cooked and showing no sign of pink.

5. Stir in the tomato sauce and ½ cup of chicken broth. Turn the heat to low and simmer for about 5 minutes.

6. Stir in the cooked rice until well combined. Remove from the heat.

7. Fill each pepper half with about ⅔ cup of filling and place them in the prepared baking dish. Top each with 1 tablespoon of Cheddar cheese.

8. Pour the remaining ½ cup of chicken broth into the bottom of the baking dish. This will help steam and soften the peppers. Tightly cover the pan with aluminum foil and bake for 45 minutes. Remove from the oven and carefully remove the foil, as steam may have become trapped in the cooking process.

PER SERVING: (2 stuffed pepper halves) Calories: 292; Total fat: 12g; Cholesterol: 62mg; Sodium: 162mg; Carbohydrates: 19g; Fiber: 3g; Protein: 23g

APRICOT CHICKEN

Fertility Booster

Prep time: 15 minutes **Cook time:** 30 minutes **Total time:** 45 minutes

Apricots are versatile and low-calorie fruits that are extremely nutritious. They possess high levels of potassium, vitamins A and C, and fiber. This flexible fruit shines equally well in sweet dishes, like your morning oats, or savory dishes, like this quick and easy chicken entrée. Serve it with a side of steamed broccoli. *Serves 4*

2 teaspoons extra-virgin olive oil

1 pound boneless skinless chicken breasts, trimmed and cut into 4 pieces

8 or 9 ripe apricots, pitted and chopped

½ cup dry white wine

½ cup low-sodium chicken broth

Juice of 1 orange

¼ cup honey

1 teaspoon dried thyme

1 tablespoon orange zest

1. In a large nonstick skillet, heat the olive oil over medium-high heat. Place the chicken breasts in the pan, cooking for 5 to 8 minutes per side, or until an instant-read thermometer indicates that their internal temperature has reached 165°F. Transfer the chicken breasts to a clean plate and cover with aluminum foil.

2. In the same skillet, combine the apricots, wine, chicken broth, orange juice, and honey. Turn the heat to high and let the liquid come to a boil. Leave the mixture uncovered, and let it boil for about 10 minutes, stirring occasionally. The sauce should be on the thick side, with the liquid reduced by half. The apricots should be broken down, but still be somewhat chunky.

3. Return the chicken to the skillet and coat with the sauce. Cook until heated through and serve.

INGREDIENT TIP: If you can't find fresh apricots, substitute an equal quantity of dried apricots. Dried apricots are a convenient source of energy, fiber, antioxidants, potassium, and iron. They can be found in most supermarkets next to other dried fruits. Purchase dried apricots that are unsweetened and sulfur free to maximize their nutritional benefits.

PER SERVING: Calories: 287; Total fat: 7g; Cholesterol: 65mg; Sodium: 49mg; Carbohydrates: 28g; Fiber: 2g; Protein: 27g

ARTICHOKE CHICKEN

Fertility Booster, Lower Calorie

Prep time: 5 minutes   **Cook time:** 35 minutes   **Total time:** 40 minutes

This dish is cheesy and decadent, but guilt free. Serve with whole-wheat pasta or a crusty whole-wheat roll. *Serves 2*

Nonstick cooking spray, for preparing the baking dish
2 boneless skinless chicken breasts
1 (14-ounce) can artichoke hearts packed in water, rinsed well and drained
1 (14.5-ounce) can no-salt-added diced tomatoes

½ cup frozen spinach, thawed and drained
½ cup dry white wine
2 slices provolone cheese
Salt-Free Italian Seasoning (page 139), for garnish (optional)

1. Preheat the oven to 375°F. Lightly coat a baking dish with cooking spray. Arrange the chicken in the baking dish.

2. Add the artichoke hearts to the chicken. Top with the tomatoes and spinach and pour the wine into the dish.

3. Cover tightly with aluminum foil and bake for 30 minutes. Uncover the dish, lay the cheese slices on top, and bake for 5 minutes more. Sprinkle with the Italian seasoning (if using).

PER SERVING: Calories: 395; Total fat: 10g; Cholesterol: 84mg; Sodium: 443mg; Carbohydrates: 30g; Fiber: 15g; Protein: 39g

CHILI-LIME CHICKEN FAJITAS WITH MANGO SALSA

Fertility Booster, Inflammation Fighter

Prep time: 20 minutes **Cook time:** 20 minutes, plus 30 minutes to chill
Total time: 1 hour, 10 minutes

Fajitas are a family favorite, and this version is quick and simple. The marinade is something you can make in just a few minutes. The mango salsa adds freshness, color, and loads of flavor while providing a boost of nutrition. Serving fajitas on corn tortillas is typically a healthier choice because corn tortillas contain whole grains and minimal ingredients. ***Serves 4***

FOR THE CHILI-LIME MARINADE

¼ cup canola oil
Zest and juice of 1 lime
2 tablespoons apple cider vinegar
1 tablespoon chili powder
1 teaspoon garlic powder
1 teaspoon onion powder
¼ teaspoon kosher salt
¼ teaspoon freshly ground black pepper

FOR THE MANGO SALSA

1 mango, peeled, pitted, and diced
½ cup fresh cilantro leaves, chopped
½ jalapeño pepper, seeded and finely minced
¼ red onion, finely diced
Zest and juice of 2 limes
¼ teaspoon kosher salt
¼ teaspoon freshly ground black pepper

FOR THE CHICKEN FAJITAS

1 pound boneless, skinless chicken breasts, cut into
 ½-inch strips
2 red bell peppers, seeded and sliced
1 red onion, sliced
8 (6-inch) corn tortillas, toasted
1 medium Hass avocado, peeled, pitted, and sliced

To make the chili-lime marinade

In a medium bowl, whisk the canola oil, lime zest and juice, vinegar, chili powder, garlic powder, onion powder, salt, and pepper until blended. Set aside.

To make the mango salsa

In a medium bowl fitted with a lid, stir together the mango, cilantro, jalapeño, red onion, lime zest and juice, salt, and pepper. Cover and refrigerate until needed.

To make the chicken fajitas

1. Add the chicken breast to the chili-lime marinade and turn to coat. Cover and refrigerate for at least 30 minutes.

2. Heat a skillet over medium heat. Add the chicken and sauté for 3 to 4 minutes until opaque.

3. Add the red bell pepper and red onion. Sauté for 3 to 4 minutes more, until the chicken is fully cooked and the vegetables are soft.

4. Scoop the chicken and vegetable mixture onto the toasted tortillas and top with the avocado and the mango salsa.

5. For leftovers, refrigerate the chicken and vegetable mixture in a microwavable airtight container for up to five days. Reheat the chicken in the microwave for 1 to 2 minutes, until heated through. Refrigerate the mango salsa in a separate airtight container for two to three days.

SUBSTITUTION TIPS: To make this vegetarian, try cubed sweet potato or low-sodium black beans instead of the chicken. You can also try pineapple, kiwi, or cantaloupe in the salsa instead of mango.

COOKING TIP: Corn tortillas are best when toasted in a dry, hot skillet on the stovetop until lightly browned on both sides.

PER SERVING: (2 tortillas) Calories: 414; Total Fat: 11g; Cholesterol: 70mg; Sodium: 458mg; Carbohydrates: 54g; Fiber: 6g; Protein: 27g

SIMPLE AND EASY LEMON BAKED COD

30-Minute, Fertility Booster, Lower Calorie

Prep time: 5 minutes **Cook time:** 15 minutes **Total time:** 20 minutes

Cod is a mild, flaky fish that is inexpensive and easy to find in most grocery stores. It is generally labeled as Atlantic or Pacific, designating the ocean from which it was caught. Atlantic and Pacific cod have the same nutritional profile, but Atlantic cod is lighter in appearance and has a slightly sweeter flavor than its more savory counterpart, Pacific-caught cod. Although not particularly high in omega-3 fatty acids, cod is still a low-fat and lean source of protein. *Serves 6*

Nonstick cooking spray, for preparing the baking dish

6 cod fillets (about 1½ pounds total), about 1 inch thick

Kosher salt

Freshly ground black pepper

2 cups cherry tomatoes

2 lemons, thinly sliced, plus more for garnish

2 tablespoons extra-virgin olive oil

2 thyme sprigs, or 1 tablespoon dried thyme

2 garlic cloves, smashed but not peeled

2 tablespoons chopped fresh parsley

1. Preheat the oven to 400°F. Lightly coat a 9-by-13-inch baking dish with cooking spray. Set aside.

2. Using a paper towel, pat the cod fillets dry. Season both sides of each fillet with salt and pepper.

3. In a medium bowl, combine the cherry tomatoes, lemon slices, olive oil, thyme, and garlic. Gently toss to mix. Pour the tomato mixture into the prepared baking dish.

4. Add the cod fillets, nestling them among the tomatoes. Bake for 15 minutes, or until the fish flakes easily with a fork.

5. Serve immediately. Garnish with parsley, fresh lemon slices, and any remaining pan sauce.

PER SERVING: Calories: 145; Total fat: 6g; Cholesterol: 49mg; Sodium: 110mg; Carbohydrates: 2g; Fiber: 1g; Protein: 20g

PISTACHIO-ENCRUSTED SALMON

30-Minute, Fertility Booster, Inflammation Fighter

Prep time: 10 minutes   **Cook time:** 14 minutes   **Total time:** 24 minutes

In addition to being loaded with heart-healthy fat, salmon is a superstar protein source. You can find it readily available in most grocery stores, and it is fast and easy to cook. Whenever possible, you should purchase wild-caught salmon. It is higher in most vitamins and minerals and lower in calories and saturated fat than farm-raised salmon because it is sourced from rivers, lakes, and oceans where it feeds on the natural habitat. It will appear bright red in color; farm-raised salmon has flesh that is more orange. *Serves 6*

6 (3-ounce) salmon fillets

⅓ cup low-fat plain Greek yogurt

⅔ cup plain whole-wheat Panko bread crumbs

⅔ cup shelled pistachios, finely chopped

½ cup minced shallot

2 tablespoons extra-virgin olive oil

2 tablespoons Dijon mustard

½ teaspoon lemon zest

¼ teaspoon red pepper flakes

1 garlic clove, minced

1. Preheat the oven to 375°F.

2. On an ungreased rimmed baking sheet, place the salmon fillets, skin-side down. Use a paper towel to pat the fish to remove any visible moisture. Use a rubber spatula to spread the Greek yogurt over each fillet.

3. In a small bowl, stir together the bread crumbs, pistachios, shallot, olive oil, Dijon mustard, lemon zest, red pepper flakes, and garlic. Put equal portions of the bread crumb mixture on top of each salmon fillet, pressing firmly so it adheres.

4. Bake for 12 to 14 minutes, or until the salmon is tender and flakes easily with a fork.

SUBSTITUTION TIP: If you like a little heat, you can swap the mustard for horseradish. Just make sure to use plain horseradish, not horseradish sauce or horseradish cream.

PER SERVING: Calories: 311; Total fat: 16g; Cholesterol: 45mg; Sodium: 274mg; Carbohydrates: 18g; Fiber: 2g; Protein: 23g

SHRIMP NOODLE BOWLS WITH GINGER BROTH

Fertility Booster, Inflammation Fighter

Prep time: 15 minutes   **Cook time:** 35 minutes   **Total time:** 50 minutes

Noodle bowls are all the rage—and for good reason. The broth here is loaded with ginger, garlic, and chili flavors. The bowls are filled with succulent shrimp, crisp vegetables, and hearty brown rice noodles. This recipe comes together quickly and is a wonderfully delicious Asian-influenced meal. *Serves 6*

1 pound shrimp, peeled and deveined, shells reserved, separated

2 cups low-sodium vegetable broth

1 (2-inch) piece fresh ginger, peeled and sliced

2 teaspoons chili-garlic sauce

¾ teaspoon kosher salt, divided

½ teaspoon freshly ground black pepper

8 ounces brown rice noodles

1 tablespoon canola oil

1 cup sugar snap peas, strings removed and thinly sliced

1 red bell pepper, seeded and thinly sliced

½ yellow onion, peeled and thinly sliced

4 garlic cloves, peeled and minced

½ cup fresh cilantro leaves (optional)

1. Place the shrimp shells in a medium pot over medium heat. Add the vegetable broth, ginger, chili-garlic sauce, ½ teaspoon of salt, and the pepper and bring to a simmer. Cook for 15 minutes.

2. While the broth simmers, bring a large pot of water to a boil over high heat. Cook the rice noodles according to the package directions. Drain and set aside.

3. In the same pot, heat the canola oil over medium heat. Add the snap peas, bell pepper, and onion. Sauté for 4 to 5 minutes until the vegetables are slightly soft.

4. Add the shrimp and cook for 2 to 3 minutes. Stir in the garlic and remaining ¼ teaspoon of salt.

5. Divide the noodles and shrimp mixture among six bowls, strain broth to remove any of the shrimp shells, and ladle into each bowl. Top with the cilantro (if using).

INGREDIENT TIPS: Chili-garlic sauce, also known as Asian chili paste or chili-garlic paste, is a staple in Asian cooking. You can often find it in the condiments aisle of your local supermarket near the soy sauce and teriyaki sauce, or in the ethnic ingredients aisle if your supermarket has one. If you can't find it, you can substitute ½ teaspoon of dried hot pepper flakes for the chili-garlic sauce. If brown rice noodles are equally difficult to find, you can use whole-grain spaghetti. And you can use chicken or salmon instead of the shrimp, if desired. Just be sure to cook the chicken to an internal temperature of 165°F.

COOKING TIP: For a richer, more flavorful broth, simmer for up to an hour.

PER SERVING: Calories: 272; Total fat: 5g; Cholesterol: 115mg; Sodium: 430mg; Carbohydrates: 36g; Fiber: 4g; Protein: 20g

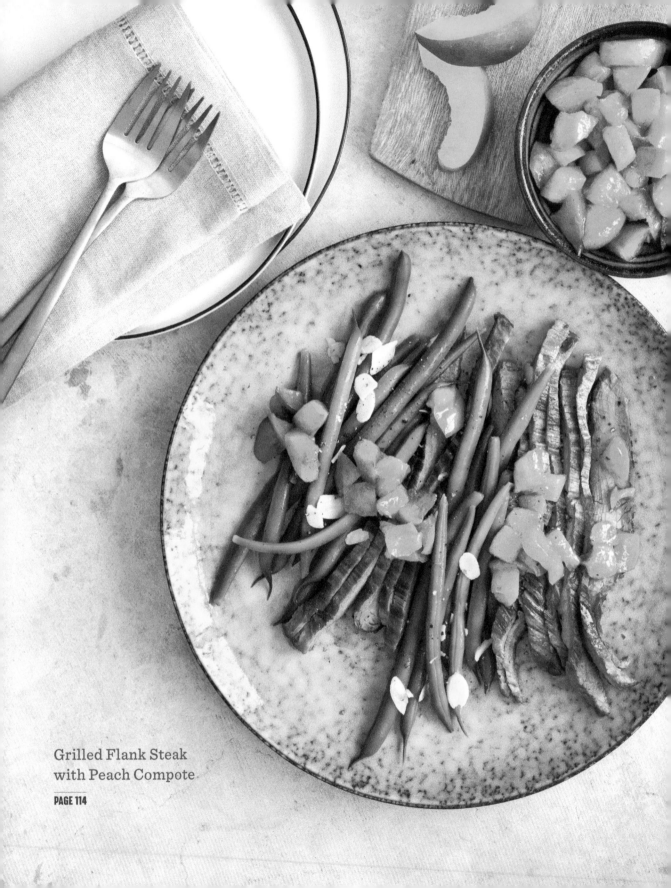

Grilled Flank Steak
with Peach Compote

PAGE 114

8.
BEEF AND PORK MAINS

SPAGHETTI SQUASH WITH MEAT SAUCE

Fertility Booster, Inflammation Fighter

Prep time: 15 minutes   **Cook time:** 1 hour, 20 minutes   **Total time:** 1 hour, 35 minutes

Spaghetti squash is a great alternative to regular pasta. With about one-fourth the calories and carbohydrates as pasta, spaghetti squash is a good source of fiber, potassium, and vitamin C. In this easy recipe, spaghetti squash is paired with carrots, celery, crushed tomatoes, and lean ground beef. It is hearty enough so you won't even miss the pasta! *Serves 6*

FOR THE SPAGHETTI SQUASH
Nonstick cooking spray, for preparing the baking sheet
2 medium spaghetti squash (about 6 pounds total)
Kosher salt
Freshly ground black pepper

FOR THE MEAT SAUCE
1 teaspoon butter
1 teaspoon extra-virgin olive oil
1½ medium carrots, chopped
1 celery stalk, finely chopped

½ cup finely chopped onion
2 garlic cloves, minced
1 pound 93% lean ground beef
Kosher salt
1 (28-ounce) can no-salt-added crushed tomatoes
¼ cup dry white wine
2 dried bay leaves
Freshly ground black pepper
6 tablespoons grated Parmesan cheese, divided

To make the spaghetti squash

1. Preheat the oven to 400°F. Coat a rimmed baking sheet with nonstick cooking spray.

2. Using a sharp knife, carefully halve the spaghetti squash vertically. Using a spoon, remove and discard the seeds and membranes. Season the flesh with salt and pepper. Place the squash halves, cut-side down, on the prepared baking sheet and bake for 1 hour, or until soft. Set aside and let cool.

To make the meat sauce

1. While the squash cooks, in a large skillet, heat the butter and olive oil over medium-low heat.

2. When the butter melts, add the carrot, celery, onion, and garlic. Sauté for 3 to 4 minutes, or until the vegetables are soft.

3. Increase the heat to medium-high and add the ground beef. Season with a pinch salt. Cook for 6 to 8 minutes, breaking up the meat with the back of a wooden spoon, or until thoroughly cooked and no pink remains. Decrease the heat to medium.

4. Add the tomatoes and wine. Simmer for about 30 minutes, or until the mixture reduces by one-fourth.

5. Cover the skillet, reduce the heat to low, and add the pepper and bay leaves. Cook for 1 hour, stirring occasionally.

6. Once the spaghetti squash is cool enough to handle, use a fork to scrape out the flesh into spaghetti-like strands. Remove the bay leaves from the sauce and discard. Portion the spaghetti squash into six shallow bowls and top each with meat sauce and 1 tablespoon of Parmesan cheese.

COOKING TIP: Pressed for time? Microwave the spaghetti squash. Halve the spaghetti squash and remove the seeds and membranes. Place the squash, cut-side down, in a microwavable dish and tightly cover with a lid or plastic wrap. Microwave on high power for 8 to 9 minutes, or until soft.

PER SERVING: Calories: 302; Total fat: 10g; Cholesterol: 54mg; Sodium: 255mg; Carbohydrates: 31g; Fiber: 8g; Protein: 21g

GRILLED FLANK STEAK WITH PEACH COMPOTE

Inflammation Fighter

Prep time: 15 minutes **Cook time:** 25 minutes **Total time:** 40 minutes

Women with PCOS may avoid red meat, believing that all of it is high in fat and unhealthy for them—but this isn't the case. Lean meats, such as flank steak, when consumed in moderation, are great sources of protein, iron, and zinc. Slice the steak against the grain and serve with a salad green for a quick and easy meal. ***Serves 6***

FOR THE PEACH COMPOTE

2 peaches, cored and diced

1 tablespoon honey

1½ teaspoons apple cider vinegar

¼ teaspoon ground cinnamon

¼ teaspoon ground ginger

¼ teaspoon ground nutmeg

¼ teaspoon kosher salt

FOR THE FLANK STEAK

1½ pounds flank steak

2 tablespoons canola oil

½ teaspoon kosher salt

¼ teaspoon freshly ground black pepper

To make the peach compote

In a small saucepan over medium heat, combine the peaches, honey, vinegar, cinnamon, ginger, nutmeg, and salt and bring to a simmer. Cook for 7 to 10 minutes, stirring frequently, until the peaches are tender, and the mixture has thickened. Remove from the heat and set aside.

To make the flank steak

1. Heat a grill to medium-high heat or place a grill pan over medium-high heat.

2. Coat the steak with the canola oil and season both sides with salt and pepper. Grill for 4 to 6 minutes per side, or until the internal temperature reaches 155°F on an instant-read thermometer.

3. Transfer to a cutting board and let rest for 5 to 10 minutes. Thinly slice the steak across the grain and serve with the peach compote.

SUBSTITUTION TIP: Try maple syrup instead of honey, if desired.

PER SERVING: Calories: 236; Total Fat: 12g; Cholesterol: 45mg; Sodium: 356mg; Carbohydrates: 7g; Fiber: 1g; Protein: 24g

ITALIAN BEEF STEW

Fertility Booster

Prep time: 15 minutes **Cook time:** 30 minutes **Total time:** 45 minutes

You can substitute ground turkey or chicken breast for the beef in this hearty stew to make it even leaner. This recipe can also be made in a slow cooker: Brown the beef and transfer it to the slow cooker with the remaining ingredients. Cover and cook on low for 6 to 8 hours. ***Serves 4***

1 pound 93% extra-lean ground beef

1 large yellow onion, chopped

3 cups sliced mushrooms

2 tablespoons minced garlic

1 tablespoon Salt-Free Italian Seasoning (page 139)

1 cup low-sodium tomato juice

1 cup brewed black coffee

¾ cup dry red wine (Cabernet or Merlot)

1 cup dry orzo

1. In a large stockpot over medium heat, combine the ground beef and onion. Cook for 7 to 8 minutes, breaking up the meat with the back of a wooden spoon, or until fully cooked and no pink remains.

2. Stir in the mushrooms, garlic, and Italian seasoning. Cook for 2 to 3 minutes, stirring occasionally.

3. Add the tomato juice, coffee, and wine. Cook until the liquid begins to simmer.

4. Add the orzo. Gently stir, cover the pot, and turn the heat to low. Simmer for 15 minutes.

> **PREPARATION TIP:** Trying to increase your fiber intake? While browning the beef, add 2 cups of carrot coins and 1 cup chopped celery and cook until softened. Want even more fiber? Swap out the orzo for an equal quantity of brown rice or quinoa (rinsed well).

PER SERVING: Calories: 399; Total Fat: 9g; Cholesterol: 80mg; Sodium: 99mg; Carbohydrates: 42g; Fiber: 3g; Protein: 30g

BEEF AND MUSHROOM STEW

Inflammation Fighter

Prep time: 20 minutes **Cook time:** 30 minutes **Total time:** 50 minutes

This beef stew has lots of ingredients, takes little effort to prepare, and is the perfect comfort food recipe. Lean beef is an excellent source of high-quality protein. When possible, do your best to seek out grass-fed beef. The nutrition of the meat you eat directly depends on the nutrition of the animal it came from. Grass-fed animals feed on grass, and so their meat is higher in antioxidants, vitamins E and A, and essential fat such as omega-3, but is lower in overall fat. Grass-fed beef may have a subtly different taste and texture because of its leanness. ***Serves 4***

1 tablespoon extra-virgin olive oil
1 teaspoon minced garlic
1 pound lean stew beef, cut into chunks
1 tablespoon apple cider vinegar
1 tablespoon low-sodium Worcestershire sauce
2 teaspoons hot sauce
1 teaspoon brown sugar
Freshly ground black pepper
1½ cups low-sodium tomato juice

1 cup Homemade Vegetable Broth (page 140), or store-bought low-sodium vegetable broth
½ cup dry red wine
1 (28-ounce) can no-salt-added diced tomatoes
3 small sweet potatoes, cut into bite-size pieces
2 cups sliced white mushrooms
1 large carrot, cut into bite-size pieces
1 cup fresh green beans, cut into 2-inch pieces
Cooked whole-wheat pasta or brown rice, for serving

1. In a large skillet, heat the olive oil and garlic over medium-high heat.

2. Add the stew beef. Sauté for 4 to 6 minutes until browned on all sides.

3. Stir in the vinegar, Worcestershire sauce, hot sauce, and brown sugar and generously season with pepper.

4. Pour in the tomato juice, vegetable broth, and wine. Reduce the heat to maintain a simmer and add the tomatoes, sweet potatoes, mushrooms, carrot, and green beans. Simmer for 20 minutes until the vegetables are tender.

5. Serve over the cooked pasta or brown rice.

> **PREPARATION TIP:** This dish can also be made in a slow cooker. After browning the beef, add all the ingredients to the slow cooker, cover, and cook on low for 6 to 8 hours.

PER SERVING: Calories: 334; Total Fat: 8g; Cholesterol: 70mg; Sodium: 253mg; Carbohydrates: 31g; Fiber: 5g; Protein: 28g

THAI PORK IN LETTUCE CUPS

Fertility Booster, Inflammation Fighter, Lower Calorie

Prep time: 40 minutes **Cook time:** 10 minutes **Total time:** 50 minutes

Lettuce wraps and PCOS go hand in hand, like peanut butter and jelly. Lettuce wraps are low in carbohydrates, and they perfectly complement any lean ground meat. We use ground pork in this recipe, but you can easily substitute lean ground beef or turkey to change up the flavor profile. These lettuce wraps are fresh, packed with tons of flavor, and easy to make. Pair this with a lightly dressed cabbage slaw and you have a winning antioxidant-packed combination. *Serves 8*

FOR THE CARROTS AND ONIONS
½ cup white vinegar
2 tablespoons sugar
⅛ teaspoon kosher salt
2 medium carrots, julienned
½ medium white onion, thinly sliced

FOR THE FILLING
1 teaspoon extra-virgin olive oil
1 pound lean ground pork
1 tablespoon peeled and minced fresh ginger
2 garlic cloves, minced
1 tablespoon low-sodium soy sauce
1 tablespoon rice vinegar

¼ teaspoon freshly ground black pepper
⅛ teaspoon kosher salt

FOR THE LETTUCE CUPS
8 Boston Bibb lettuce leaves
½ English cucumber, chopped
1 small jalapeño pepper, seeded and finely minced
1 cup chopped scallion
½ cup fresh basil, finely chopped
½ cup fresh cilantro, hard stems removed and finely chopped
½ cup fresh mint, finely chopped
¼ cup unsalted raw peanuts, chopped
Lime wedges, for serving

To make the carrots and onions

In a small bowl, whisk the vinegar, sugar, and salt until well blended. Stir in the carrots and onion and let marinate at room temperature for 30 minutes.

To make the filling

1. In a large skillet, heat the olive oil over medium heat.

2. Add the ground pork, ginger, and garlic. Cook for 7 to 9 minutes, or until the pork is no longer pink, breaking up any large pieces of pork with the back of a wooden spoon. Drain the excess liquid and oil off the pork and discard.

3. Stir in the soy sauce, vinegar, pepper, and salt.

CONTINUED >>

To assemble the lettuce cups

1. Drain the excess liquid off the carrot-onion mixture.

2. Place ⅛ of the cooked pork mixture into each lettuce leaf. Top each pork and lettuce cup with equal parts cucumber, jalapeño, scallion, and carrot-onion mixture.

3. Sprinkle with basil, cilantro, mint, and peanuts. Serve with the lime wedges to squeeze over the top of each lettuce cup. Fold the lettuce over the filling and consume immediately.

PER SERVING: (1 lettuce cup) Calories: 199; Total fat: 11g; Cholesterol: 38mg; Sodium: 312mg; Carbohydrates: 12g; Fiber: 2g; Protein: 13g

GRILLED PORK AND PINEAPPLE KEBABS

Fertility Booster, Inflammation Fighter

Prep time: 20 minutes **Cook time:** 20 minutes **Total time:** 40 minutes

Kebabs are a traditional summer treat, and this version gets a sweet upgrade with fresh pineapple, red bell pepper, and a mixture of honey, soy sauce, and apple cider vinegar. If you have a bit of extra time, marinate the kebabs first, but they're equally delicious brushed with the sauce while grilling. ***Serves 6***

2 pounds pork tenderloin, cubed

1 small pineapple, peeled, cored, and cubed (about 3 cups)

2 red bell peppers, seeded and cut into 2-inch pieces

1 red onion, peeled and cut into 2-inch pieces

¾ teaspoon kosher salt, divided

½ teaspoon freshly ground black pepper, divided

1½ tablespoons canola oil

1 tablespoon honey

1½ teaspoons low-sodium soy sauce

1½ teaspoons apple cider vinegar

1½ teaspoons ground cumin

1. Preheat the grill to medium heat, or place a grill pan over medium heat.

2. While the grill warms, thread the cubed pork, pineapple, red bell peppers, and red onion onto skewers, alternating the ingredients. Season the kebabs with half the salt and half the pepper.

3. In a small bowl, whisk together the canola oil, honey, soy sauce, vinegar, cumin, and the remaining salt and pepper. Brush half the marinade onto the kebabs.

4. Grill the kebabs for 3 to 4 minutes per side, or until the pork reaches 145°F on an instant-read thermometer and the vegetables are tender. Each time you flip the kebabs, brush with additional marinade.

SUBSTITUTION TIP: For a vegetarian version, substitute cubed tofu for the pork tenderloin.

COOKING TIP: If using wooden skewers, soak them in water for 30 minutes before threading the pork and vegetables to keep the skewers from charring or catching on fire.

PER SERVING: Calories: 381; Total Fat: 14g; Cholesterol: 119mg; Sodium: 423mg; Carbohydrates: 17g; Fiber: 2g; Protein: 45g

GRILLED PORK TENDERLOIN WITH GARLIC AND HERBS

5-Ingredient, Fertility Booster, Lower Calorie

Prep time: 10 minutes **Cook time:** 1 hour, plus 15 minutes to rest **Total time:** 1 hour, 25 minutes

Pork tenderloin is always a showstopper when entertaining. Because it's so low in fat, you'll need to stuff it full of garlic and herbs to flavor the meat as it cooks. Good news: You'll have plenty of those flavorful leftovers to tuck into sandwiches and to dress up salads for the rest of the week. *Serves 6*

1 (3-pound) pork tenderloin
2 tablespoons extra-virgin olive oil
4 garlic cloves, minced

2 tablespoons chopped fresh thyme leaves
4 or 5 small rosemary sprigs

1. Preheat a grill to medium-high heat, or place a grill pan over medium-high heat.

2. Make an incision about 1-inch deep along the entire length of the fatty side of the tenderloin. Rub the tenderloin with the olive oil, including inside the cut.

3. Pack the incision with the garlic, thyme, and rosemary and pinch it shut. Grill the pork for 1 hour, turning it every 15 minutes, or until the internal temperature registers 145°F on an instant-read thermometer.

4. Let the tenderloin rest for 15 minutes before slicing and serving.

PER SERVING: Calories: 285; Total Fat: 13g; Cholesterol: 130mg; Sodium: 131mg; Carbohydrates: 1g; Fiber: 0g; Protein: 40g

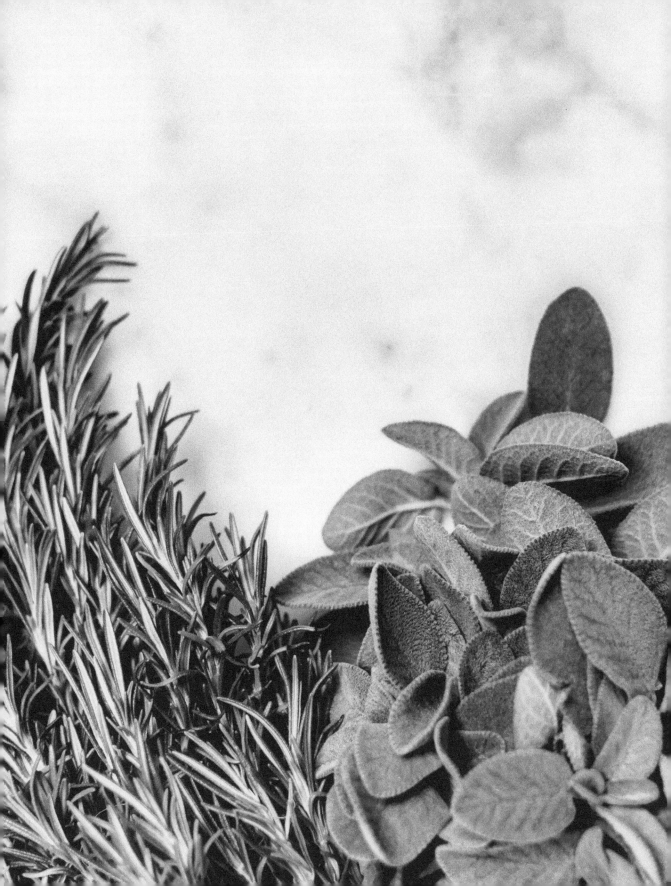

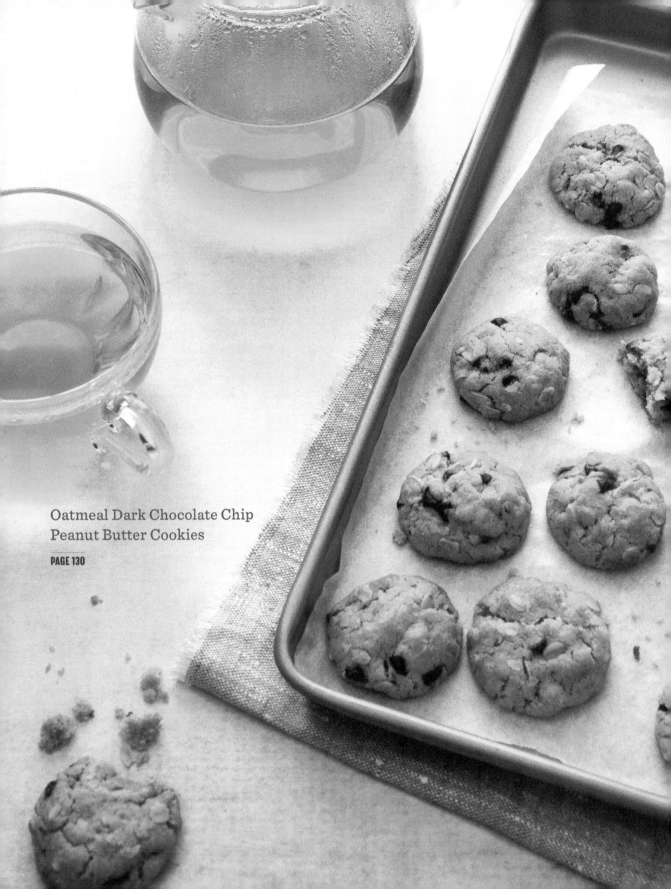

Oatmeal Dark Chocolate Chip
Peanut Butter Cookies

PAGE 130

9.
SNACKS, SIDES, AND DESSERTS

PORTOBELLO MUSHROOMS WITH RICOTTA, TOMATO, AND MOZZARELLA

5-Ingredient, 30-Minute, Fertility Booster, Inflammation Fighter, Lower Calorie

Prep time: 5 minutes   **Cook time:** 20 minutes   **Total time:** 25 minutes

These deliciously topped mushrooms make a healthy appetizer, or a tasty side dish when paired with Fennel-Apple-Walnut Salad (page 75) or Simple and Easy Lemon Baked Cod (page 106). *Serves 6*

6 portobello mushroom caps, stemmed, gills removed

1 tablespoon extra-virgin olive oil

1½ cups part-skim ricotta, divided

3 small Roma tomatoes, thinly sliced

¾ cup shredded part-skim mozzarella cheese

1. Preheat the oven to 400°F. Line a baking sheet with parchment paper or aluminum foil.

2. Clean any debris from the outer mushroom caps with a damp paper towel. Rub the inner and outer portions of the mushroom caps with olive oil and place them, top-side down, on the prepared baking sheet.

3. Spread ¼ cup of ricotta over the inside of each mushroom cap. Top each mushroom cap with tomato slices and sprinkle with about 1 tablespoon of mozzarella cheese.

4. Bake for 15 to 20 minutes, or until the cheese turns golden brown. Serve immediately.

PER SERVING: (1 mushroom cap) Calories: 176; Total fat: 10g; Cholesterol: 36mg; Sodium: 271mg; Carbohydrates: 10g; Fiber: 2g; Protein: 12g

PINTO BEAN–STUFFED SWEET POTATOES

Fertility Booster, Inflammation Fighter

Prep time: 15 minutes   **Cook time:** 45 minutes to 1 hour   **Total time:** 1 hour, 15 minutes

This recipe can do double duty as a hearty side dish or as a light lunch or dinner when paired with a side salad. ***Serves 6***

6 medium sweet potatoes, scrubbed and patted dry

1 (16-ounce) can low-sodium pinto beans, rinsed well and drained

3 medium tomatoes, seeded and diced

1 tablespoon extra-virgin olive oil

1½ teaspoons ground cumin

1½ teaspoons ground coriander

⅛ teaspoon kosher salt

1 cup low-fat plain Greek yogurt, divided

1. Preheat the oven to 400°F. Line a rimmed baking sheet with aluminum foil.

2. Using a fork, prick the outside of each sweet potato in about 5 or 6 different places. Place the sweet potatoes on the prepared baking sheet and bake for about 45 minutes to 1 hour, depending on size. Remove from the oven and set aside.

3. In a small saucepan over medium heat, combine the pinto beans, tomatoes, olive oil, cumin, coriander, and salt. Cook for 3 to 4 minutes until warm, then remove from the heat.

4. When the sweet potatoes are cool enough to handle, halve each sweet potato lengthwise. Using a metal spoon, gently press down on the flesh of the potato, creating a small well. Fill the well with the bean-tomato mixture and top each with about 2 tablespoons of yogurt.

PER SERVING: (2 potato halves) Calories: 227; Total fat: 2g; Cholesterol: 2mg; Sodium: 234mg; Carbohydrates: 42g; Fiber: 7g; Protein: 11g

ROASTED VEGETABLES

30-Minute, Fertility Booster, Inflammation Fighter, Lower Calorie

Prep time: 15 minutes **Cook time:** 15 minutes **Total time:** 30 minutes

This is a colorful, nutrient-packed side dish brimming with fiber and antioxidants. Higher-fiber foods can help combat insulin resistance by slowing how quickly the body releases insulin and blood sugar. Antioxidants are especially important for women with PCOS as they help decrease a woman's risk of inflammation and other chronic diseases. ***Serves 6***

Nonstick cooking spray, for preparing the baking sheet

2 tablespoons extra-virgin olive oil

4 garlic cloves, minced

½ teaspoon Salt-Free Italian Seasoning (page 139)

2 cups fresh broccoli florets

1 zucchini, cut into 1-inch coins

1 yellow squash, sliced and quartered

1 red bell pepper, membranes removed, cut into ½-inch strips

1 medium red onion, quartered

Kosher salt

Freshly ground black pepper

1. Preheat the oven to 425°F. Coat a rimmed baking sheet with cooking spray. Set aside.

2. In a large bowl, whisk together the olive oil, garlic, and Italian seasoning.

3. Add the broccoli, zucchini, yellow squash, red bell pepper, and red onion. Gently toss to coat.

4. Spread the vegetable mixture on the prepared baking sheet. Roast for 13 to 16 minutes, or until tender. Season with salt and pepper.

COOKING TIP: Baking time may vary depending on the size of your vegetables.

VARIATION TIP: Experiment with seasonal vegetables and different spices to add a whole new dimension to this recipe.

PER SERVING: Calories: 88; Total fat: 5g; Cholesterol: 0mg; Sodium: 19mg; Carbohydrates: 10g; Fiber: 3g; Protein: 3g

GREEN BEANS WITH TOASTED ALMONDS

30-Minute, Fertility Booster, Inflammation Fighter, Lower Calorie

Prep time: 5 minutes **Cook time:** 10 to 15 minutes **Total time:** 20 minutes

The toasted almonds add heart-healthy fat, flavor, and crunch to this side dish. ***Serves 6***

1½ pounds fresh green beans, trimmed

2 tablespoons extra-virgin olive oil

2 teaspoons butter

½ cup slivered almonds

1 garlic clove, minced

2 tablespoons freshly squeezed lemon juice

Kosher salt

Freshly ground black pepper

1. Fill a 6-quart pot with 2 inches of water and bring it to a boil over high heat. Add the green beans and boil for 2 minutes, or until crisp-tender. In a large colander, drain and rinse the green beans under cold running water until completely cool. Place the green beans on a clean kitchen towel and gently pat.

2. In a large skillet, heat the olive oil and butter over medium-low heat until the butter melts and the foam subsides.

3. Stir in the almonds and toast for about 3 minutes, stirring occasionally, until they're golden brown, making sure they do not burn. Using a slotted spoon or metal spatula, transfer the almonds to a plate to cool.

4. Decrease the heat under the skillet to low and add the garlic. Cook, stirring constantly, for 1 minute. Increase the heat to medium and add the green beans. Cook for 4 to 7 minutes, tossing frequently, until the green beans become lightly browned in places.

5. Add the lemon juice and toss to mix. Season with salt and pepper. Transfer to a serving dish and sprinkle with the toasted almonds.

PER SERVING: Calories: 117; Total fat: 7g; Cholesterol: 3mg; Sodium: 19mg; Carbohydrates: 9g; Fiber: 3g; Protein: 3g

HONEY-ROASTED SUNFLOWER AND PUMPKIN SEEDS

30-Minute, Fertility Booster, Inflammation Fighter

Prep time: 5 minutes   **Cook time:** 15 minutes   **Total time:** 20 minutes

These nutritious seeds are delicious as a snack or on top of a soup or salad. ***Serves 12***

1½ cups raw unsalted sunflower seeds

1½ cups raw unsalted pumpkin seeds

2 tablespoons honey

2 tablespoons extra-virgin olive oil

½ teaspoon ground cinnamon

⅛ teaspoon kosher salt

1. Preheat the oven to 325°F. Line a rimmed baking sheet with parchment paper. Set aside.

2. In a medium bowl, combine the sunflower seeds, pumpkin seeds, honey, olive oil, cinnamon, and salt. Toss well.

3. Arrange the seeds in a single layer on the prepared baking sheet. Bake for 15 minutes, stirring once halfway through the baking time, until lightly browned.

4. Let cool to room temperature. Refrigerate in an airtight container where the seeds can keep for up to two weeks in the refrigerator. They can also be frozen and will last up to three months when stored in an airtight container in the freezer.

PER SERVING: (¼ cup) Calories: 220; Total fat: 18g; Cholesterol: 54mg; Sodium: 29mg; Carbohydrates: 9g; Fiber: 4g; Protein: 8g

BALSAMIC BERRIES AND RICOTTA

30-Minute, Fertility Booster, Inflammation Fighter, Lower Calorie

Prep time: 10 minutes **Total time:** 10 minutes

Any type of berry will do in this easy and refreshing dessert! ***Serves 2***

¼ cup balsamic vinegar

1 tablespoon loosely packed brown sugar

1 teaspoon vanilla extract

½ cup fresh strawberries, sliced

½ cup fresh raspberries

½ cup fresh blackberries

½ cup part-skim ricotta

1. In a medium bowl, whisk the vinegar, brown sugar, and vanilla until well combined.

2. Add the strawberries, raspberries, and blackberries. Gently toss to coat. Marinate the fruit for 15 minutes. Drain and discard the marinade.

3. To serve, divide the ricotta between two small dishes and top each with half the berry mixture.

PER SERVING: Calories: 165; Total fat: 5g; Cholesterol: 19mg; Sodium: 63mg; Carbohydrates: 21g; Fiber: 5g; Protein: 9g

OATMEAL DARK CHOCOLATE CHIP PEANUT BUTTER COOKIES

30-Minute, Lower Calorie

Makes 24 cookies **Prep time:** 15 minutes **Cook time:** 10 minutes **Total time:** 25 minutes

These cookies include wholesome ingredients such as peanut butter, rolled oats, and dark chocolate chips. Bake them for 8 minutes for a chewier cookie, or for 10 minutes for a crispier cookie. For a fluffier cookie, refrigerate the dough for 30 minutes before baking. Any way you decide to make them, they'll be the perfect guilt-free dessert.

1½ cups natural creamy peanut butter

½ cup packed dark brown sugar

2 large eggs

1 cup old-fashioned rolled oats

1 teaspoon baking soda

½ teaspoon kosher salt

½ cup dark chocolate chips

1. Preheat the oven to 350°F. Line a baking sheet with parchment paper. Set aside.
2. In the bowl of a stand mixer fitted with the paddle attachment, whip the peanut butter until very smooth.
3. Continue beating and add the brown sugar, mixing until combined.
4. One at a time, add the eggs, beating the first one until fluffy before adding the next.
5. Mix in the oats, baking soda, and salt until combined.
6. Using a rubber spatula, fold in the chocolate chips by hand.
7. Using a small cookie scoop or teaspoon, place small portions of cookie dough on the prepared baking sheet about 2 inches apart. Bake for 8 to 10 minutes, depending on your preferred level of doneness.

INGREDIENT TIP: If you need (or prefer) to make a gluten-free version of these cookies, simply use gluten-free oats.

VARIATION TIP: Try raisins instead of chocolate chips.

PER SERVING: (1 cookie) Calories: 152; Total fat: 10g; Cholesterol: 18mg; Sodium: 131mg; Carbohydrates: 12g; Fiber: 2g; Protein: 4g

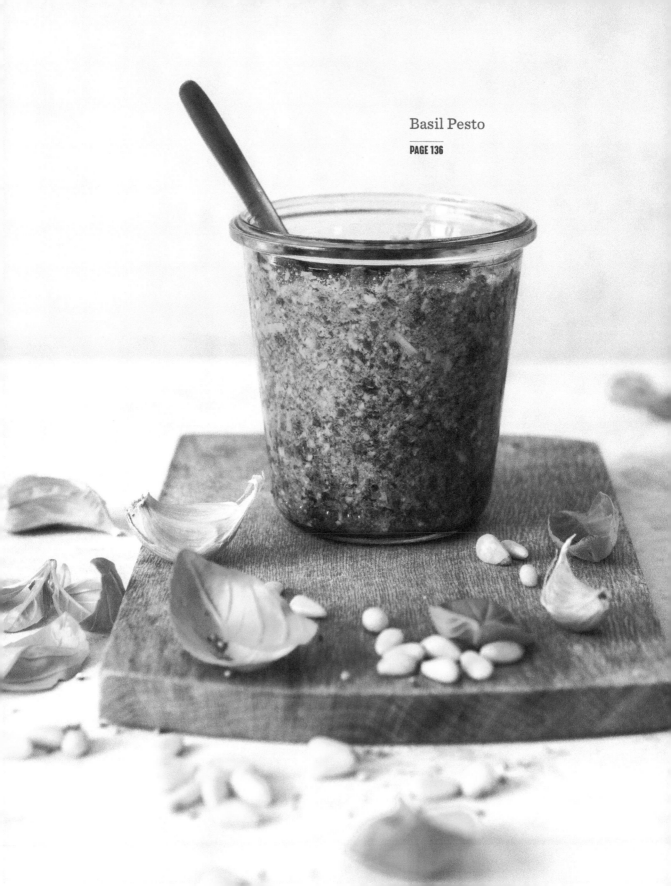

Basil Pesto

PAGE 136

10.
KITCHEN STAPLES, CONDIMENTS, AND SAUCES

SIMPLE VINAIGRETTE

Lower Calorie

Makes ½ cup   Prep time: 5 minutes, plus 30 minutes to chill   **Total time:** 35 minutes

This light and refreshing salad dressing also goes great with greens and vegetables. Change up the flavor by using different vinegars and seasonings.

½ cup red wine vinegar

⅓ cup extra-virgin olive oil

1 tablespoon freshly squeezed lemon juice

1 tablespoon Salt-Free Italian Seasoning (page 139)

1 garlic clove, crushed

⅛ teaspoon ground white pepper

In a small bowl, whisk the vinegar, olive oil, lemon juice, Italian seasoning, garlic, and white pepper. Cover and refrigerate for at least 30 minutes before serving.

PER SERVING: (2 teaspoons) Calories: 60; Total fat: 6g; Cholesterol: 0mg; Sodium: 15mg; Carbohydrates: 0g; Fiber: 0g; Protein: 0g

BALSAMIC VINAIGRETTE

30-Minute, Inflammation Fighter, Lower Calorie

Makes about ¾ cup Prep time: 5 minutes **Total time:** 5 minutes

This is an easy, versatile dressing that can double as both a salad dressing and a marinade. You can control the sodium count by adjusting the amount of salt you add. This vinaigrette is so flavorful, you may not need any salt at all!

¾ cup extra-virgin olive oil

¼ cup balsamic vinegar

½ cup diced shallot

1 garlic clove, minced

1 tablespoon Dijon mustard

Kosher salt

Freshly ground black pepper

In a blender, combine the olive oil, vinegar, shallot, garlic, and mustard. Blend until smooth. Season with salt and pepper. Cover and refrigerate for up to seven days.

PER SERVING: (2 teaspoons) Calories: 65; Total fat: 7g; Cholesterol: 0mg; Sodium: 15mg; Carbohydrates: 1g; Fiber: 0g; Protein: 0g

BASIL PESTO

30-Minute

Makes 3½ cups **Prep time:** 10 minutes **Total time:** 10 minutes

Pesto is a quintessential Northern Italian sauce and condiment that features fresh basil. Not only is it delicious, it is considered heart-healthy because it's made with the superfoods olive oil, nuts, and garlic. A little goes a long way, though, as it's loaded with flavor but is also calorie dense.

1 cup fresh basil leaves

1 cup fresh baby spinach leaves

½ cup freshly grated Parmesan cheese

½ cup extra-virgin olive oil

¼ cup pine nuts

4 garlic cloves, peeled

¼ teaspoon kosher salt, plus more as needed

¼ teaspoon freshly ground black pepper, plus more as needed

1. In a food processor, combine the basil, spinach, Parmesan cheese, olive oil, pine nuts, garlic, salt, and pepper. Process until a paste forms, stopping to scrape down the sides of the bowl with a spatula, as needed. Taste, and adjust the seasoning if necessary.

2. Refrigerate in an airtight container for up to five days, or freeze the pesto in an airtight container for up to two months and thaw as needed. Or divide the pesto into ice cube trays, seal in a plastic bag, and freeze for up to two months. Pop the handy pesto cubes out of the tray as needed.

VARIATION TIP: Try any nuts, like pepitas, walnuts, or almonds instead of pine nuts, if desired.

PER SERVING: (½ cup) Calories: 209; Total fat: 20g; Cholesterol: 0mg; Sodium: 231mg; Carbohydrates: 2g; Fiber: 1g; Protein: 4g

HOMEMADE HUMMUS

30-Minute, Inflammation Fighter, Lower Calorie

Prep time: 10 minutes **Total time:** 10 minutes

Hummus can be used as an ingredient in a sandwich such as the Vegetable and Hummus Pita (page 83) or served straight up with raw vegetables for a simple, healthy snack. ***Serves 6***

1 (16-ounce) can reduced-sodium chickpeas, rinsed well and drained, with ½ cup liquid reserved

3 tablespoons freshly squeezed lemon juice

2 tablespoons extra-virgin olive oil

3 garlic cloves, minced

¼ teaspoon freshly ground black pepper

¼ teaspoon ground cumin

¼ teaspoon paprika

1. In a food processor or blender, purée the chickpeas.

2. Add the lemon juice, olive oil, garlic, pepper, cumin, and paprika. Blend well to combine.

3. Add the reserved liquid, 1 to 2 tablespoons at a time, blending until smooth. Serve immediately, or cover with plastic wrap and refrigerate for 3 to 5 days.

PER SERVING: (¼ cup) Calories: 101; Total fat: 5g; Cholesterol: 0mg; Sodium: 85mg; Carbohydrates: 13g; Fiber: 4g; Protein: 4g

HOMEMADE BEANS

5-Ingredient, Fertility Booster, Inflammation Fighter, Lower Calorie

Makes 5 to 6 cups **Prep time:** 2 hours **Cook time:** 1 hour **Total time:** 3 hours

Beans are a staple on the DASH diet. Although all the recipes in this book use low sodium beans, when you make them from scratch you control the amount of salt added. This recipe can be made with any type of dried beans. The sodium content will vary with the amount of salt you add as seasoning.

1 pound dried beans, any kind

2 dried bay leaves

Kosher salt

Freshly ground black pepper

1. Lay out the beans on a rimmed sheet pan. Look through them carefully and discard any small stones or debris. Rinse well.

2. In a large soup pot, combine the dried beans with enough cold water to cover them completely (3 to 4 inches of water usually does the trick). Cover the pot and bring it to a boil. Allow the beans to boil for 1 minute. Remove the pot from the stove and set it aside, keeping the cover on, for 1 hour.

3. Drain the beans and rinse out the pot. Place the beans back into the clean pot and add the bay leaves. Cover with 2 inches of cold water and bring to a boil over high heat. Skim off and discard any thin film that develops on the water as the beans boil.

4. Reduce the heat. Simmer the beans for 1 to 1½ hours, or until tender. Remove and toss the bay leaves. Season with salt and pepper.

PER SERVING: (½ cup cooked beans) Calories: 115; Total fat: 1g; Cholesterol: 0mg; Sodium: 5mg; Carbohydrates: 20g; Fiber: 7g; Protein: 8g

SALT-FREE ITALIAN SEASONING

30-Minute, Lower Calorie

Makes about ½ cup **Prep time:** 5 minutes **Total time:** 5 minutes

¼ cup dried basil

3 tablespoons dried oregano

3 tablespoons dried parsley flakes

2 tablespoons garlic powder

1 teaspoon dried thyme

1 teaspoon dried rosemary, crushed

¼ teaspoon freshly ground black pepper

⅛ teaspoon red pepper flakes

In a small airtight container with a lid, combine the basil, oregano, parsley, garlic powder, thyme, rosemary, black pepper, and red pepper flakes. Cover and shake vigorously to combine. Keep stored in an airtight container for up to six months.

PER SERVING: (¼ teaspoon) Calories: 1; Total fat: 0g; Cholesterol: 0mg; Sodium: 0mg; Carbohydrates: 1g; Fiber: 0g; Protein: 0g

HOMEMADE VEGETABLE BROTH

Inflammation Fighter, Lower Calorie

Makes about 6 cups **Prep time:** 10 minutes **Cook time:** 45 minutes **Total time:** 55 minutes

Making your own vegetable broth is a great way to save money and recycle your vegetable scraps. By saving and freezing the tops, skins, bottoms, and any other vegetable pieces you would ordinarily discard, you are left with the foundation for a healthy, homemade low-sodium vegetable broth.

1 tablespoon extra-virgin olive oil

2 large onions, roughly chopped

4 garlic cloves, chopped

4 celery stalks, chopped

4 large carrots, scrubbed clean and chopped

About 8 cups water (you may need more depending on the amount of vegetable scraps)

Frozen vegetable scraps (at least 3 cups)

3 dried bay leaves

Fresh herbs of choice, such as thyme, parsley, basil, oregano

Kosher salt

Freshly ground black pepper

1. In a large stockpot, warm the olive oil over medium heat. Add the onions and garlic and cook for 1 to 2 minutes until the onions are translucent. Add the celery and carrots and cook for 5 to 7 minutes more, until softened, stirring often to prevent sticking. Add the water, frozen vegetable scraps, bay leaves, and fresh herbs. Season with salt and pepper.

2. Decrease the heat to low and partially cover the pot. Simmer for at least 45 minutes.

3. Place a colander or mesh strainer over a large pot. Pour the broth through the strainer. Discard the vegetables and herbs, reserving just the broth. Use the broth immediately or transfer to an airtight container and refrigerate for up to five days, or freeze for up to three months.

PER SERVING: (1 cup) Calories: 25; Total fat: 0g; Cholesterol: 0mg; Sodium: 0mg; Carbohydrates: 1g; Fiber: 0g; Protein: 0g

PCOS DIARY: TRACK YOUR REACTIONS

THE DIRTY DOZEN™ AND THE CLEAN FIFTEEN™

A nonprofit environmental watchdog organization called Environmental Working Group (EWG) looks at data supplied by the US Department of Agriculture (USDA) and the Food and Drug Administration (FDA) about pesticide residues. Each year it compiles a list of the best and worst pesticide loads found in commercial crops. You can use these lists to decide which fruits and vegetables to buy organic to minimize your exposure to pesticides and which produce is considered safe enough to buy conventionally. This list does not mean these fruits and vegetables are pesticide free, though, so wash these fruits and vegetables thoroughly. The list is updated annually, and you can find it online at EWG.org/FoodNews.

Dirty Dozen™

1. Strawberries
2. Spinach
3. Kale
4. Nectarines
5. Apples
6. Grapes
7. Peaches
8. Cherries
9. Pears
10. Tomatoes
11. Celery
12. Potatoes

Additionally, nearly three-fourths of hot pepper samples contained pesticide residues.

Clean Fifteen™

1. Avocados
2. Sweet Corn*
3. Pineapples
4. Sweet Peas (Frozen)
5. Onions
6. Papayas*
7. Eggplants
8. Asparagus
9. Kiwis
10. Cabbages
11. Cauliflower
12. Cantaloupes
13. Broccoli
14. Mushrooms
15. Honeydew Melons

* A small amount of sweet corn, papaya, and summer squash sold in the United States is produced from genetically modified seeds. Buy organic varieties of these crops if you want to avoid genetically modified produce.

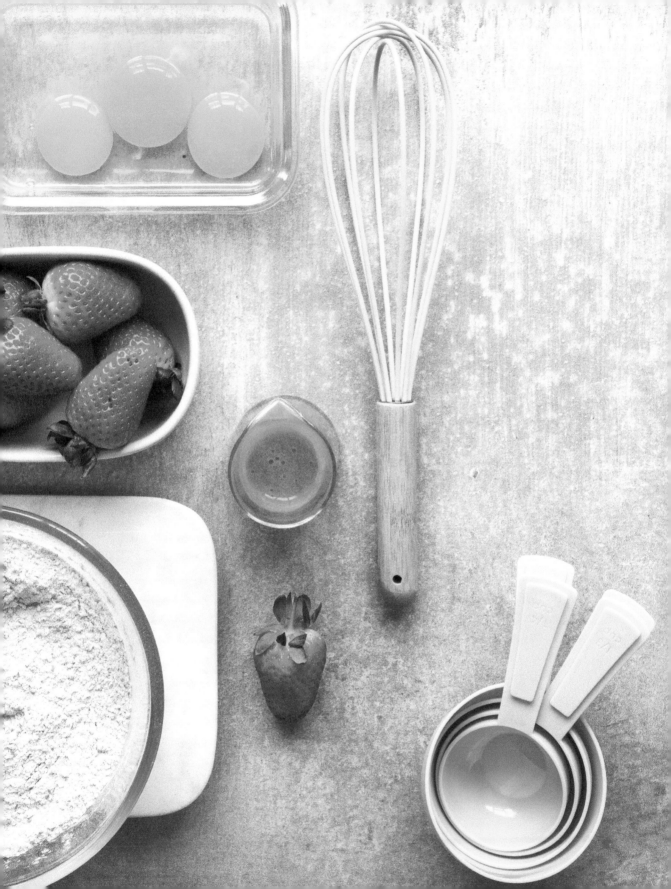

MEASUREMENT CONVERSIONS

VOLUME EQUIVALENTS (LIQUID)

US STANDARD	US STANDARD (OUNCES)	METRIC (APPROXIMATE)
2 tablespoons	1 fl. oz.	30 mL
¼ cup	2 fl. oz.	60 mL
½ cup	4 fl. oz.	120 mL
1 cup	8 fl. oz.	240 mL
1½ cups	12 fl. oz.	355 mL
2 cups or 1 pint	16 fl. oz.	475 mL
4 cups or 1 quart	32 fl. oz.	1 L
1 gallon	128 fl. oz.	4 L

OVEN TEMPERATURES

FAHRENHEIT	CELSIUS (APPROXIMATE)
250°F	120°C
300°F	150°C
325°F	165°C
350°F	180°C
375°F	190°C
400°F	200°C
425°F	220°C
450°F	230°C

VOLUME EQUIVALENTS (DRY)

US STANDARD	METRIC (APPROXIMATE)
⅛ teaspoon	0.5 mL
¼ teaspoon	1 mL
½ teaspoon	2 mL
¾ teaspoon	4 mL
1 teaspoon	5 mL
1 tablespoon	15 mL
¼ cup	59 mL
⅓ cup	79 mL
½ cup	118 mL
⅔ cup	156 mL
¾ cup	177 mL
1 cup	235 mL
2 cups or 1 pint	475 mL
3 cups	700 mL
4 cups or 1 quart	1 L

WEIGHT EQUIVALENTS

US STANDARD	METRIC (APPROXIMATE)
½ ounce	15g
1 ounce	30g
2 ounces	60g
4 ounces	115g
8 ounces	225g
12 ounces	340g
16 ounces or 1 pound	455g

REFERENCES

Andersen, Per, Ingeborg Seljeflot, Michael Abdelnoor, Herald Arnesen, Per Olva Dale, Astrid Lovik, Kare Birkeland, et al. "Increased Insulin Sensitivity and Fibrinolytic Capacity After Dietary Intervention in Obese Women with Polycystic Ovary Syndrome." *Metabolism* 44, no. 5 (1995): 611–6.

Appel, L. J., M. W. Brands, S. R. Daniels, N. Karanja, P. J. Elmer, and F. M. Sacks. "Dietary Approaches to Prevent and Treat Hypertension: A Scientific Statement from the American Heart Association." *Hypertension* 47, no. 2 (2006): 296–308.

Ard, J. D., S. C. Grambow, D. Liu, C. A. Slentz, W. E. Kraus, and L. P. Svetkey. "The Effect of the PREMIER Interventions on Insulin Sensitivity." *Diabetes Care* 27 (2004): 340–7.

Asemi, Zatollah, Mansooreh Samimi, Zohreh Tabassi, Hossein Shakeri, Sima-Sadat Sabihi, and Ahmad Esmaillzadeh. "Effects of DASH Diet on Lipid Profiles and Biomarkers of Oxidative Stress in Overweight and Obese Women with Poly-cystic Ovary Syndrome: A Randomized Clinical Trial." *Nutrition* 30, nos. 11-12 (November-December 2014): 1287–93. doi:10.1016/j.nut.2014.03.008.

Azziz, R., E. Carmina, D. Dewailly, E. Diamanti-Kandarakis, H. F. Escobar-Morreale, W. Futterweit, O. E. Janssen, et al. "Positions Statement: Criteria for Defining Poly-cystic Ovary Syndrome as a Predominantly Hyperandrogenic Syndrome: An Androgen Excess Society Guideline." *The Journal of Clinical Endocrinology & Metabolism* 91, no. 11 (November 2006): 4237–45.

Centers for Disease Control and Prevention. "High Blood Pressure Fact Sheet." Accessed on May 8, 2019: https://www.cdc.gov/dhdsp/data_statistics/fact_sheets/fs_bloodpressure.htm.

Ciaraldi, T. P., A. el-Roeiy, Z. Madar, D. Reichart, J. M. Olefsky, and S. S. Yen. "Cellular Mechanisms of Insulin Resistance in Polycystic Ovarian Syndrome." *The Journal of Clinical Endocrinology & Metabolism* 75, no. 2 (August 1, 1992): 577–83. doi.org/10.1210/jcem.75.2.1322430.

Corbould, Anne, Young-Bum Kim, Jack F. Youngren, Celia Pender, Barbara B. Kahn, Anna Lee, and Andrea Dunaif. "Insulin Resistance in the Skeletal Muscle of Women with PCOS Involves Intrinsic and Acquired Defects in Insulin Signaling." *American Journal of Physiology: Endocrinology and Metabolism* 288, no. 5 (2005): E1047–54. doi.org/10.1152/ajpendo.00361.2004.

Dantas, Wagner Silva, Bruno Gualano, Michele Patrocínio Rocha, Cristiano Roberto Grimaldi Barcellos, Viviane dos Reis Vieira Yance, and José Antonio Miguel Marcondes. "Metabolic Disturbance in PCOS: Clinical and Molecular Effects on Skeletal Muscle Tissue." *The Scientific World Journal*, vol. 2013, Article ID 178364 (2013). doi:10.1155/2013/178364.

Diamanti-Kandarakis, E., and A. Papavassiliou. "Molecular Mechanisms of Insulin Resistance in Polycystic Ovary Syndrome." *Trends in Molecular Medicine* 12, no. 7 (2006): 324–32.

Diamanti-Kandarakis E., and C. D. Christakou. "Insulin Resistance in PCOS." In *Diagnosis and Management of Polycystic Ovary Syndrome*, eds. Farid, N. R., and E. Diamanti-Kandarakis. Boston, MA: Springer, 2009.

Douglas, C. C., B. A. Gower, B. E. Darnell, F. Ovalle, R. A. Oster, and R. Azziz. "Role of Diet in the Treatment of Polycystic Ovary Syndrome." *Fertility and Sterility* 85, no. 3 (2006): 679–88. doi:10.1016/j.fertnstert.2005.08.045.

Drosdzol, Agnieszka, Violetta Skrzypulec, Barbara Mazur, Romana Pawlińska-Chmara, Duleba A. J., and A. Dokras. "Quality of Life and Marital Sexual Satisfaction in Women with Polycystic Ovary Syndrome." *Folia Histochemica et Cytobiologica* 45, Supplement 1 (2007): S93–7.

Duleba, A. J., and A. Dokras. "Is PCOS an Inflammatory Process?" *Fertility and Sterility* 97, no. 1 (2012): 7–12. doi:10.1016/j.fertnstert.2011.11.023.

Dunaif, A. "Insulin Resistance and the Polycystic Ovary Syndrome: Mechanism and Implications for Pathogenesis." *Endocrine Reviews* 18, no. 6 (1997): 774–800.

Eisenberg, S. "Looking for the Perfect Brew." *Science News* 133, no. 16 (1988): 252–3.

Elsenbruch, Sigrid, Susanne Hahn, Daniela Kowalsky, Alexandra H. Öffner, Manfred Schedlowski, Klaus Mann, Onno E. Janssen, et al. "Quality of Life, Psychosocial Well-Being, and Sexual Satisfaction in Women with Polycystic Ovary Syndrome." *The Journal of Clinical Endocrinology & Metabolism* 88 (2003): 5801–7.

Feldeisen, S., and K. Tucker. "Nutritional Strategies in the Prevention and Treatment of Metabolic Syndrome." *Applied Physiology, Nutrition, and Metabolism* 32, no. 1 (2007): 46–60.

Fernandez, R. C., V. M. Moore, E. M. Van Ryswyk, T. J. Varcoe, R. J. Rodgers, W. A. March, L. J. Moran, J. C. Avery, R. D. McEvoy, and M. J. Davies. "Sleep Disturbances in Women with Polycystic Ovary Syndrome: Prevalence, Pathophysiology, Impact and Management Strategies." *Nature and Science of Sleep* 10 (2018): 45–64. doi:10.2147/NSS.S127475.

Garg, D., and R. Tal. "Inositol Treatment and ART Outcomes in Women with PCOS." *International Journal of Endocrinology*. 2016 (2016): 1979654. doi:10.1155/2016/1979654.

Gaskins, A. J., and J. E. Chavarro. "Diet and Fertility: A Review." *American Journal of Obstetrics & Gynecology* 218, no. 4 (2018): 379–89. doi:10.1016/j.ajog.2017.08.010.

Gierisch, Jennifer M., Remy R. Coeytaux, Rachel Peragallo Urrutia, Laura J. Havrilesky, Patricia G. Moorman, William J. Lowery, Michaela Dinan, et al. "Oral Contraceptive Use and Risk of Breast, Cervical, Colorectal, and Endometrial Cancers: A Systematic Review." *Cancer Epidemiology, Biomarkers & Prevention* 22, no. 11 (2013): 1931–43.

Günalan, E., A. Yaba, and B. Yılmaz. "The Effect of Nutrient Supplementation in the Management of Polycystic Ovary Syndrome–Associated Metabolic Dysfunctions: A Critical Review." *Journal of the Turkish-German Gynecological Association* 19, no. 4 (2018): 220–32. doi:10.4274/jtgga.2018.0077.

Hahn, Susanne, Onno E. Janssen, Susanne Tan, Katja Pleger, Klaus Mann, Manfred Schedlowski, Rainer Kimmig, Sven Benson, Efthimia Balamitsa, and Sigrid Elsenbruch. "Clinical and Psychological Correlates of Quality-Of-Life in Polycystic Ovary Syndrome." *European Journal of Endocrinology* 153, no. 6 (2005): 853–60.

Hinderliter, A. L., M. A. Babyak, A. Sherwood, and J. A. Blumenthal. "The DASH Diet and Insulin Sensitivity." *Current Hypertension Reports* 13, no. 1 (2011): 67–73. doi:10.1007/s11906-010-0168-5.

Hirschberg, A. L., S. Naessén, M. Stridsberg, B. Byström, and J. Holte. "Impaired Cholecystokinin Secretion and Disturbed Appetite Regulation in Women with Polycystic Ovary Syndrome." *Gynecological Endocrinology* 19, no. 2 (2004): 79–87, doi:10.1080/09513590400002300.

Institute of Medicine (IOM). Food and Nutrition Board. *Dietary Reference Intakes: Calcium, Phosphorus, Magnesium, Vitamin D, and Fluoride.* Washington, DC: National Academy Press, 1997.

Kelly, Chris C., Helen Lyall, John R. Petrie, Gwyn W. Gould, John M. C. Connell, and Naveed Sattar. "Low Grade Chronic Inflammation in Women with Polycystic Ovarian Syndrome." *The Journal of Clinical Endocrinology & Metabolism* 86, no. 6 (2001): 2453–5.

Kloss, J. D., M. L. Perlis, J. A. Zamzow, E. J. Culnan, and C. R. Gracia. "Sleep, Sleep Disturbance, and Fertility in Women." *Sleep Medicine Reviews* 22 (2015): 78–87. doi:10.1016/j.smrv.2014.10.005.

Krystock, Amy. "Role of Lifestyle and Diet in the Management of Polycystic Ovarian Syndrome." In *Polycystic Ovary Syndrome*, ed. Pal, Lubna. New York, NY: Springer, 2014.

Liese, Angela D., Michele Nichols, Xuezheng Sun, Ralph B. D'Agostino, and Steven M. Haffner. "Adherence to the DASH Diet Is Inversely Associated with Incidence of Type 2 Diabetes: The Insulin Resistance Atherosclerosis Study." *Diabetes Care* 32, no. 8 (2009): 1434–6. doi:10.2337/dc09-0228.

López-García E., R. M. van Dam, T. Y. Li, F. Rodriguez-Artalejo, and F. B. Hu. "The Relationship of Coffee Consumption with Mortality." *Annals of Internal Medicine* 148, no. 12 (2008): 904–14.

Markopoulos, M. C., G. Valsamakis, E. Kouskouni, A. Boutsiadis, I. Papassotiriou, G. Creatsas, and G. Mastorakos. "Study of Carbohydrate Metabolism Indices and Adipocytokine Profile and Their Relationship with Androgens in Polycystic Ovary Syndrome After Menopause." *European Journal of Endocrinology* 168, no. 1 (2013): 83–90.

McGrice, M., and J. Porter. "The Effect of Low-Carbohydrate Diets on Fertility Hormones and Outcomes in Overweight and Obese Women: A Systematic Review." *Nutrients* 9, no. 3 (2017): 204. doi:10.3390/nu9030204.

McRae, M. P. "Dietary Fiber Intake and Type 2 Diabetes Mellitus: An Umbrella Review of Meta-analyses." *Journal of Chiropractic Medicine* 17, no. 1 (2018): 44–53. doi:10.1016/j.jcm.2017.11.002.

Michels, K. A., R. M. Pfeiffer, L. A. Brinton, and B. Trabert. "Modification of the Associations Between Duration of Oral Contraceptive Use and Ovarian, Endometrial, Breast, and Colorectal Cancers." *JAMA Oncology* 4, no. 4 (2018): 516–21. doi:10.1001/jamaoncol.2017.4942.

Monash University. "International Evidence-Based Guideline for the Assessment and Management of Polycystic Ovary Syndrome (PCOS)." www.monash.edu/medicine/sphpm/mchri/pcos/guideline. Accessed May 21, 2019.

Murri, M., M. Luque-Ramırez, M. Insenser, M. Ojeda-Ojeda, and H. F. Escobar-Morreale. "Circulating Markers of Oxidative Stress and Polycystic Ovary Syndrome (PCOS): A Systematic Review and Meta-analysis." *Human Reproduction Update* 19, no. 3 (2013): 268–88.

National Heart, Lung, and Blood Institute. "Your Guide to Lowering Your Cholesterol with Therapeutic Lifestyle Changes." https://www.nhlbi.nih.gov/health-topics/all-publications-and-resources/your-guide-lowering-cholesterol-therapeutic-lifestyle. Accessed June 11, 2019.

Panth, N., A. Gavarkovs, M. Tamez, and J. Mattei. "The Influence of Diet on Fertility and the Implications for Public Health Nutrition in the United States." *Frontiers in Public Health* 6 (2018): 211. doi:10.3389/fpubh.2018.00211.

Pliquett, R. U., D. Führer, S. Falk, S. Zysset, D. Y. von Cramon, and M. Stumvoll. "The Effects of Insulin on the Central Nervous System—Focus on Appetite Regulation." *Hormone and Metabolic Research* 38, no. 7 (2006): 442–6. doi:10.1055/s-2006-947840.

Raja-Khan, N., K. Agito, J. Shah, C. M. Stetter, T. S. Gustafson, H. Socolow, A. R. Kunselman, D. K. Reibel, and R. S. Legro. "Mindfulness-based Stress Reduction for Overweight/Obese Women with and without Polycystic Ovary Syndrome: Design and

Methods of a Pilot Randomized Controlled Trial." *Contemporary Clinical Trials* 41 (2015): 287–97. doi:10.1016/j.cct.2015.01.021.

Randeva, H. S., B. K. Tan, M. O. Weickert, K. Lois, J. E. Nestler, N. Sattar, and H. Lehnert. "Cardiometabolic Aspects of the Polycystic Ovary Syndrome." *Endocrine Reviews* 33, no. 5 (2012): 812–41.

Romualdi, Daniela, Valentina Immediata, Simona De Cicco, Valeria Tagliaferri, and Antonio Lanzone. "Neuroendocrine Regulation of Food Intake in Polycystic Ovary Syndrome." *Reproductive Sciences* 25, no. 5 (2018): 644–53.

Sharifi, Faranak, Sahar Mazloomi, Reza Hajihosseini, and Saideh Mazloomzadeh. "Serum magnesium concentrations in polycystic ovary syndrome and its association with insulin resistance." *Gynecological Endocrinology* 28, no. 1 (2012): 7–11. doi:10.3109/09513590.2011.579663.

Shetty, Disha, Baskaran Chandrasekaran, Arul Watson Singh, and Joseph Oliverraj. "Exercise in Polycystic Ovarian Syndrome: An Evidence-Based Review." *Saudi Journal of Sports Medicine* 17, no. 3 (2017): 123–28.

Shin, C. S., and K. M. Kim. "The Risks and Benefits of Calcium Supplementation." *Endocrinology and Metabolism* (Seoul) 30, no. 1 (2015): 27–34. doi:10.3803/EnM.2015.30.1.27.

Soltani, S., F. Shirani, M. J. Chitsazi, and A. Salehi-Abargouei. "The Effect of Dietary Approaches to Stop Hypertension (DASH) Diet on Weight and Body Composition in Adults: A Systematic Review and Meta-Analysis of Randomized Controlled Clinical Trials." *Obesity Reviews* 17, no. 5 (2016): 442–54. doi: 10.1111/obr.12391.

Sonoma Press. *The DASH Diet for Beginners: The Guide to Getting Started.* Berkeley, CA: Arcas Publishing, 2014.

Stepto, N. K., S. Cassar, A. E. Joham, S. K. Hutchison, C. L. Harrison, R. F. Goldstein, and H. J. Teede. "Women with Polycystic Ovary Syndrome Have Intrinsic Insulin Resistance on Euglycaemic-Hyperinsulaemic Clamp." *Human Reproduction* 28, no. 3 (2013): 777–84.

Suri, J., J. C. Suri, B. Chatterjee, P. Mittal, and T. Adhikari. "Obesity May Be the Common Pathway for Sleep-Disordered Breathing in Women with Polycystic Ovary Syndrome." *Sleep Medicine* 23 (2016): 32–9.

Trent, M. E., M. Rich, S. B. Austin, and C. M. Gordon. "Quality of Life in Adolescent Girls with Polycystic Ovary Syndrome." *Archives of Pediatrics and Adolescent Medicine* 156, no. 6 (2002): 556–60.

Tsilchorozidou, Tasoula, John W. Honour, and Gerard S. Conway. "Altered Cortisol Metabolism in Polycystic Ovary Syndrome: Insulin Enhances 5Alpha-Reduction But Not the Elevated Adrenal Steroid Production Rates." *The Journal of Clinical Endocrinology & Metabolism* 88, no. 12 (2003): 5907–13. doi:10.1210/jc.2003-030240.

Unfer, V., J. E. Nestler, Z. A. Kamenov, N. Prapas, and F. Facchinetti. "Effects of Inositol(s) in Women with PCOS: A Systematic Review of Randomized Controlled Trials." *International Journal of Endocrinology* 2016 (2016): 1849162. doi:10.1155/2016/1849162.

Unluturk, U., A. Harmanci, C. Kocaefe, and B. O. Yildiz. "The Genetic Basis of the Polycystic Ovary Syndrome: A Literature Review Including Discussion of PPAR-gamma." *PPAR Research* 2007 (2007): 49109. doi:10.1155/2007/49109.

U.S. Department of Health and Human Services and U.S. Department of Agriculture. *Dietary Guidelines for Americans 2015-2020.* 8th ed. Washington, D.C.: U.S. Department of Health and Human Services, 2015. http://www.health.gov/dietaryguidelines/2015. Accessed June 11, 2019.

Whelton, P. K., J. He, L. J. Appel, J. A. Cutler, S. Havas, T. A. Kotchen, E. J. Roccella, et al. "Primary Prevention of Hypertension: Clinical and Public Health Advisory from the National High Blood Pressure Education Program." *JAMA* 288, no. 15 (2002): 1882–8.

Wild, R. A. "Long-term Health Consequences of PCOS." *Human Reproduction Update* 8, no. 3 (2002): 231–41.

Xue, B., A. G. Greenberg, F. B. Kraemer, and M. B. Zemel. "Mechanism of Intracellular Calcium ($[Ca^{2+}]_i$) Inhibition of Lipolysis in Human Adipocytes." *The FASEB Journal* 15 (2001): 2527–9.

RESOURCES

Harvard Health Publishing: www.health.harvard.edu

Harvard Health Publishing is an informative website that offers comprehensive educational materials on health- and wellness-related topics. Search the term "anti-inflammatory foods" on the website's search engine and you will find various educational resources related to the topic.

Mayo Clinic: www.mayoclinic.org

Here you'll find a wealth of material on the DASH diet—everything from sample meal plans to shopping tips and helpful guidelines on how to stick to the DASH diet when dining out. Enter "DASH diet" into the search line on the main site to access a wide variety of information.

National Heart, Lung, and Blood Institute: www.nhlbi.nih.gov/health-topics /dash-eating-plan

This website is a great resource for learning more about the traditional DASH diet eating plan and its numerous health benefits.

The PCOS Dietitian: www.thepcosdietitian.com

My website contains helpful dietary and lifestyle resources for women with PCOS.

Soul Cysters: www.soulcysters.com

Soul Cysters is the largest online community of women with PCOS. On their website they feature personal stories, book recommendations, recipes, videos, and information about getting a proper diagnosis. The community is active with social media on the following outlets:

Facebook: PCOS - SoulCysters.com

Instagram: PCOS_Soulcyster

Pinterest: PCOSSoulcyster

YouTube: PCOS SoulCyster

Taste of Home: www.tasteofhome.com/collection/dash-diet-recipes

The website for the magazine *Taste of Home* offers a variety of DASH-friendly recipes in their article "60 Recipes to Jump Start the DASH Diet." Although women with PCOS need to be mindful of their overall carbohydrate intake when following the DASH diet, the recipes listed here are sure to spark some inspiration.

INDEX

ACKNOWLEDGMENTS

Without the help, support, and encouragement from many notable people, this book would never have come to fruition. First and foremost, I would like to thank the team at Callisto Media for trusting my expertise as a PCOS nutrition expert to write on such an important, worthwhile topic. My editor, Marisa Hines, made a challenging project appear seamless, and I thank you, Marisa, for your guidance, upbeat attitude, and professionalism. I also want to thank Mary Cassells, my development editor, for your thoughtful feedback, careful eye, and attention to detail in completing my edits. I feel extremely fortunate and blessed to have had the fortune to work with an awesome rock-star writing team.

I would also like to thank my mentors, Dr. Pal and Dr. Kodaman at Yale Fertility and Endocrinology. The PCOS community is so lucky to have such wonderful physicians dedicated to the health and wellness of their patients. I could not be more appreciative of your endless support of my practice. It means the world to me that you trust me with your patients and I am forever grateful.

To the fabulous dietitians at The Plano Program: Audrey Castell-Watts, RD, and Emily Gerdner, RD, LDN, CDE—whether or not you realize it, you helped make this book happen. Without question, you both "stepped up to the plate" by taking on a larger patient load so I could dedicate my time to writing. I can't thank you both enough for being the fabulous dietitians that you are and for strengthening our field one patient at a time.

To my patients struggling with PCOS, you are the ultimate inspiration for this book. There is not one day that goes by that I don't think about your struggles and how I can make it easier for you. Your stories, personal anecdotes, and triumphs are forever inspiring, and the main reason I continue to search for the best dietary solutions and strategies to help you thrive. I thank you for your courage, perseverance, and bravery, which motivates me every day to go to work.

Finally, to my sweet, sweet husband, Marc. Truly, without you this book would have never happened. From day one of our relationship you have always challenged me to follow my dreams. Whenever I start to doubt myself you are everlastingly my biggest cheerleader. You push me to be a better version of me. Thank you for allowing me to make room in our busy life to complete this project.

ABOUT THE AUTHOR

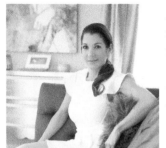

Amy Plano is an author, wellness activist, professor, wife, foodie, and registered dietitian specializing in the unique nutritional needs of women with PCOS. Let's get real. Having PCOS is hard. Managing all the not-so-fun symptoms that come along with the disorder is even harder. That's where Amy comes in.

For more than 10 years, Amy has been working closely with the top doctors in women's health and fertility to design the most comprehensive and effective nutrition programs for women with PCOS. Through her research and clinical work, she has learned what works and what does not work.

Amy offers a variety of services for women with PCOS, ranging from free educational content, mind-blowing blog posts, and sassy videos on her fabulous website (www.thepcosdietitian.com) to one-on-one nutritional counseling sessions and customized meal plans. Amy's mission is to educate, inspire, and motivate women with PCOS so they can be the healthiest and happiest versions of themselves.